LIZZIE WEBB'S
TOTAL HEALTH & FITNESS

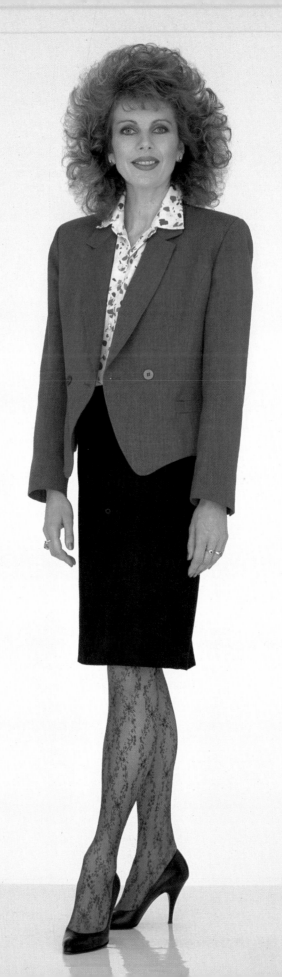

LIZZIE WEBB'S
TOTAL HEALTH & FITNESS

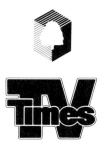

First published in 1989 by Boxtree Limited
Published in association with Independent
Television Books Ltd.

British Library Cataloguing in Publication Data
Webb, Lizzie
Lizzie Webb's total health & fitness
1. Physical fitness
I. Title
613.7

ISBN 1-85283-271-1

Special Photography by Harry Ormesher
Make-up Mandy Asquith
Hairdresser Ken Devonshire

The publishers gratefully acknowledge the help of
the following companies: British American Tobacco
Co UK (p 106); Clarins & Wella; TV Times (pp 20,
21, 33, 34, 37, 43, 45, 46); Sea Fish Industry
Authority (pp 18, 29, 38, 41, 44); Summer Orange
Office (pp 23, 27); Fresh Fruit and Vegetable
Information Bureau (pp 48, 51, 53, 55)

Design: Bob Gordon
Editor: Susie Ward
Managing Editor: Anna Selby

Typeset by Florencetype Ltd, Kewstoke, Avon
Printed and bound in Belgium by
Proost International Book production
for Boxtree Limited
36 Tavistock Street
London WC2E 7PB

CONTENTS

INTRODUCTION

Live life to the full – no matter what age you are!
Why feel bloated, overweight, tired and depressed
when the *quality* of your life can so
easily be transformed. Everything you need to
know about total fitness and feeling good (let alone
looking a million dollars) is here in this book. Our
motto is 'Be fit on the inside and the outside and put
a spring in your step for the rest of your life'.
Look forward from now on to feeling on top
of the world – it's down to you – with a little
help from me!

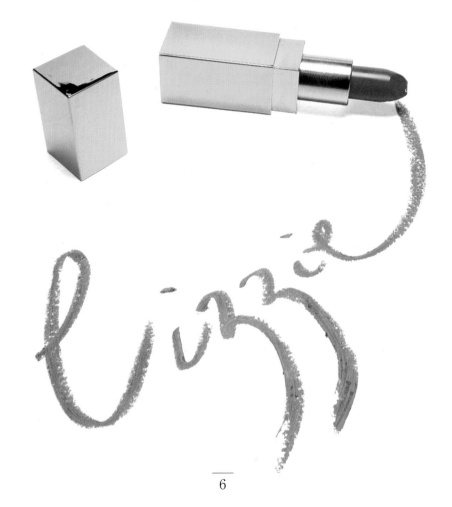

TOTAL HEALTH & FITNESS

FOOD and DRINK

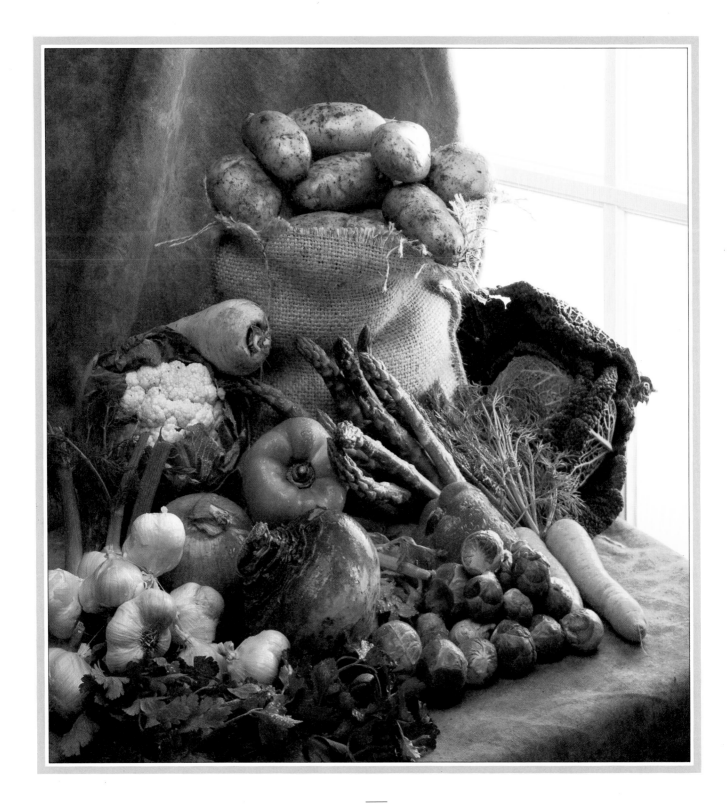

the HEALTHY HAPPY EATER

At last the parade of superstars plugging their 'secret' solutions to weight loss, eternal youth and drop-dead good looks has moved off centre stage. Public disillusion has hastened the eclipse. Some of the personalities themselves have provided unhappy proof of what can happen when stress and temptation take over where the much-publicised diet leaves off, while the thousands – sometimes millions – who bought their books have come to realise that the

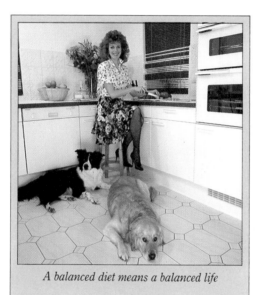

A balanced diet means a balanced life

Hollywood way to fitness is a career in itself, a course in self-absorption and physical management that only those who are paid to pursue it can afford, either in terms of time or money.

At the same time, 'real' people have also become aware that fad and fashion diets don't deal with the basic problem most of us face: to eat healthily *and* enjoyably *all* the time, while maintaining a sensible weight. Some 35% of us weigh over 10% more than we should – for a woman of average height and build that could mean anything from 12lb to 3 or more stone. As for the remaining 65%, most will insist that an

extra 6 to 10lbs is hanging unwanted somewhere around the hips, thighs or tummy. When we do make up our minds to lose the excess, however, we tend to sacrifice long-term benefits for short-term success: our aim is to get to our target weight as quickly as possible.

Impatience is the curse of our day and age. Speed is of the essence, especially when it comes to losing weight. Everyone wants results *now*. Excess weight saps confidence and can even depress, so an attack on fat is as much for our spirit as for physical appearance. And the sooner we feel better, the better we feel.

What this rush to a newer, more gorgeous you fails to accept is that you can't keep up the pace forever. You are pitting the stamina of a sprinter against the rigours of a cross-country race. And as in the fable, it's slow and steady who wins, by turning the race into a life-long commitment to good eating and good health.

So keep your expectations high, but change emphasis. The best way to improve your figure is to improve your eating habits. And to regard a slim figure not mainly as a source of more compliments, but as an investment in a longer, healthier life. Remember, there is no such thing as bad food – only bad diets.

LOOKING GOOD IS FEELING GOOD

Nutritionists and doctors agree that the food we eat has an enormous amount to do with the way we look and feel. It affects us directly – a balanced diet means we have the necessary energy to carry on living life to the full. It shows in the clearness of our skin, the brightness of our eyes and the shine of our hair – assets that become more and more valuable when you no longer have the simple attraction of youth on your side. The general consensus of modern medical opinion is that a lower intake of fats, less cholesterol and more fibre in our diets lowers the risk of heart disease, stroke, high blood pressure, arthritis, gall stones, ulcers, constipation and even, perhaps, certain cancers. There is also evidence to suggest that a diet higher in fruits and vegetables and lower in red meats and animal protein can reduce stress and slow down the ageing process.

That is not to say that to get the best results you must be a strict vegetarian but, based on contemporary research, a move toward that direction makes sense. Studies of vegetarian groups have revealed that they suffer less from heart disease, strokes and gallstones. Some American analyses have indicated that their average life span may be as much as 10 years longer than that of meat eaters *and* they spend less time in hospital. They also look leaner and fitter – have you ever seen a fat vegetarian? So even if you can't see yourself cutting out the pleasures of meat entirely, steer toward poultry and fish rather than steak, lamb and pork, increase your intake of wholegrain cereal foods

– such as wholemeal bread, brown rice and pasta – as well as potatoes and pulses, and cut way down on foods which are high in animal fat and/or sugar. Personally, I don't even eat chicken; I prefer my protein to come from eggs, fish and cheese – but that is a personal choice based on my own unhappiness at the way we raise animals for slaughter. I have included poultry recipes in this book, since I know that many people do not share my feelings, and that a healthy source of nutrients should not be lightly eliminated. In following my ideology, I realize that balance is very important: eggs, shellfish and cheese are all high in cholesterol, so I don't overdo my love of all three.

As you can see, I'm not a fanatic when it comes to eating healthily – I *enjoy* my food. But I am sensible enough to realise that if I make an effort to understand what different foods actually contain, it will help my body share the benefits of my enjoyment. That knowledge enables you to plan your diet so that the balance of complex carbohydrates, fibre, unsaturated fats, animal and vegetable protein is kept at the maximum level for health and energy, as well as good looks. Let's take a short refresher course in nutrition:

Carbohydrates and Fibre
Carbohydrates include four broad food categories which we commonly call sugars, starches, fibre and alcohol. Of these, the most important to a healthy diet are starches and fibre. Most starch and fibre sources come largely under the heading of complex carbohydrates – now known to be as important as protein to a healthy diet. Cereals and root vegetables make the largest contribution, and are most often cooked to aid digestion. However, we should strive to include a greater variety of complex carbohydrates in our meals; more grains, pulses, vegetables and fruit on a daily basis. In addition we should eat

them raw, or as lightly cooked as possible, to conserve the high ratio of vitamins, minerals and plant protein.

Certain types or parts of complex carbohydrates are indigestible: they form the fibre which adds bulk to food. Although fibre has no positive food value, it plays an important role in maintaining a healthy digestive tract, aiding in the passage of waste and the elimination of fat and poisonous chemicals which cause constipation, inflammation of the colon and worse.

The refined carbohydrates – white flour, rice and pasta – should be replaced by wholemeal versions. Because they are more slowly metabolised, unrefined foods supply a steady stream of energy throughout the day. They keep us satisfied longer, thus preventing between-meal snacking and overeating. As for refined sugar – cut it out, as much as you can. Satisfy your sweet tooth with *natural* sugar – fructose – from fruit and berries.

And alcohol? Well, the golden rule is a little, not too often. Stick to wine; a glass of white has between 80–90 calories. It's really the calorie content which should make you careful – and the knowledge that a steady stream of alcohol acts much like caffeine in coffee, slowing down the action of the liver and thus, our metabolic rate. Remember, our whole aim is to have the most energetic system possible!

Cholesterol

This is one of the more confusing constituents of our diet. In fact, cholesterol is essential for life. It is naturally made in our own bodies, and is also contained in the animal-derived foods we eat. If all goes well, our own production of cholesterol should decrease in relation to the amount we take in from outside. But with our increased intake of animal fat in the last couple of generations, our bodies' capacity to adapt has often broken down and the cholesterol level has

---

TIPS FOR *HEALTHY SHOPPING, COOKING AND EATING*

○ All fish is nutritious, but white fish has even less fat than the oily varieties such as mackerel, herring or sardines.

○ If you are eating canned fish, always drain thoroughly. Try to use fish packed in brine or tomato sauce rather than in vegetable oil.

○ Remove the skin from chicken and poultry before eating it, if it has not been removed before cooking (it is often kept on during cooking to impart flavour). You will save about 20 calories an ounce.

○ If you are eating meat, trim off all visible fat before cooking – and before eating, if you are at a restaurant.

○ If a recipe calls for cream, try substituting low-calorie yoghurt or 1% fromage frais. Sometimes there is no substitute – but then use as little as possible or go without!

○ Try not to peel vegetables whenever possible; simply wash and scrub them. Eat vegetables raw as often as possible. When you do cook, only do so until they are tender-crisp – never until soft (unless you are making a purée!).

○ Use non-stick frying pans and saucepans as often as possible. While butter or oil must be used for sautéeing, you can use low-fat and dairy spreads for sauces and oven-roasting.

○ Grill, bake or steam whenever you have the option. These are the three best ways to preserve nutrients and lose fat.

○ Try beginning meals with a first course of fruit – grilled grapefruit, sliced peaches with cottage cheese – or a salad of tomatoes or greens. Cut down your main course proportionally. It's a neat cheat for filling up – and cutting down on calories.

---

simply risen higher in many individuals. This high level is a primary risk in heart disease, since excess cholesterol builds up a sticky silt-like deposit in the arteries, impeding the passage of blood and increasing the pressure on the heart.

The highest proportion of cholesterol is found in egg yolk, offal, shellfish, red meat, butter and cream. Since most of these foods (except shellfish) are also high in fat, it is a doubly-good reason to decrease their dominance of our diet.

Fats – Saturated and Unsaturated

All major dietary guidelines advocate a need to reduce our average national fat consumption. As of 1987, 38% of our daily energy (kilocalorie) intake has been calculated as fat. The National Advisory Council on Nutritional Education has targeted 30% as the optimum level for health, while several doctors would advise an even lower rate. This conscious decrease should apply to both saturated and unsaturated fats.

Weight for weight, fat has almost twice as many calories as sugar and, while some fat is necessary to supply the body with a ready source of energy, there is no doubt that we rely too much on it, to the detriment of healthier foods such as the complex carbohydrates. While we absorb about the same amount of protein as fat, it is the fat which causes the biggest problem to the figure-conscious, since it stores more efficiently, becoming even harder to shift. The biggest villain is that ad man's bug-bear 'saturated fat' – found in meats, oily fish and dairy products.

As a rule, the harder a fat is at room temperature, the more saturated it is. Suet, and fat on chops and steaks, contains around 60% saturated fat, while butter contains some 50%. Polyunsaturated margarines and low-fat margarines are not totally without saturated fat – 15–12% is usual – while polyunsaturated oils are 12% and below. In addition to the weight we gain from careless reliance on fatty foods, it also contributes to high cholesterol levels (see above). As for polyunsaturated fats, these are a preferable substitute in our diet, but even they should not be regarded as totally beneficial. While a reasonable level of polyunsaturates have been shown to lower harmful cholesterol levels in the blood, an excess of polyunsaturates has also been linked to tumours in rats, though no trials have proved a similar link in humans.

All polyunsaturated oils have the same number of calories – 120 per tablespoon – but they vary in their saturation levels. Best for slimmers are corn, safflower and grape oils – generic 'vegetable oil' is the highest. Olive oil is a monosaturate, and as such was once discriminated against by weight-watchers and nutrition gurus, even though it too contained only 120 calories per tablespoon. New evidence suggests, however, that it has an important part to play in the lowering of harmful cholesterol.

Protein

After World War II the catchword for a newly health-conscious society was 'protein'. Plenty of meat, eggs, and dairy products were prescribed – even bread was 'protein-enriched'.

Certainly protein is necessary to life. It is converted by our digestive tract into amino acids, which in turn are transformed into another form of protein which powers our systems. It is necessary for cell and tissue renewal, and children need a steady supply for growth, but the emphasis on the importance of animal protein in our diet has been grossly exaggerated. It has reached the point that our enthusiastic consumption has become more of a risk than an asset.

Today we British eat almost twice the recommended daily amount of protein-rich food – our intake is 100–110g, instead of the safer 56g. Because it is the most complex of all food elements, protein is the hardest to break down

TOP LOW-CALORIE FOODS

All-Bran (per 50g/20z serving)	140 calories	Lettuce (per medium head)	15 calories
Apple (medium)	45 calories	Melon (average 175g/6oz slice)	25 calories
Apricot (per fruit)10 calories		Milk (skimmed, per 120ml/¼pt)	50 calories
Aubergine (medium 200g/7oz)	30 calories	Mushrooms (100g/4oz raw)	40 calories
Banana (medium)	80 calories	Mussels (per mussel)	10 calories
Bean sprouts (50g/2oz serving)	20 calories	Nectarine (per average fruit)	75 calories
French beans (100g/4oz serving)	7 calories	Onion (per 75g/3oz onion)	20 calories
Runner beans 100g/4oz serving)	20 calories	Orange (per average 150g/5oz fruit)	35 calories
Haricot beans (75g/3oz serving)	90 calories	Peach (per average 100g/4oz fruit)	35 calories
Baked beans in tomato sauce		Pear (per average 100g/4oz fruit)	35 calories
(per 200g/7oz can)	140 calories	Pears (per average 100g/4oz serving)	60 calories
Beetroot (per baby beet)	5 calories	Green or red pepper	
Bread (wholemeal slice)	60–70 calories	(per 150g/5oz pepper)	20 calories
Brussels sprouts (per sprout)	5 calories	Pineapple (average fresh ring)	25 calories
Cabbage (100g/4oz serving)	20 calories	Plaice (steamed fillet – 150g/5oz)	125 calories
Carrots (per 50g/2oz serving)	20 calories	Plum (average 35g/1½oz fruit)	15 calories
Cauliflower (per 100g/4oz serving)	13 calories	Potato (baked, 200g/7oz potato)	175 calories
Edam cheese (per 25g/1oz slice)	90 calories	Prawns (with shell – per 25g/1oz)	10 calories
Low-calorie cottage cheese		Prawns (shelled – per 25g/1oz)	30 calories
(per 100g/4oz serving)	80 calories	Sole (steamed – 150g/5oz fillet)	125 calories
Chicken (roast, no skin		Spinach (steamed or lightly boiled –	
– per 150g/5oz piece)	125 calories	100g/4oz serving)	50 calories
Cod (per 150g/5oz piece)	125 calories	Tangerine (per 75g/3oz fruit)	35 calories
Corn on the cob (average cob)	85 calories	Tomato (per 50g/2oz fruit)	10 calories
Crab (white meat –		Trout (steamed 175g/6oz trout	
75g/3oz serving)	105 calories	on bone)	125 calories
Cucumber (per 100g/4oz piece)	10 calories	Tuna (canned in brine –	
Egg (large, size 2)	90 calories	90g/3½oz can)	105 calories
Endive or chicory (75g/3oz serving)	15 calories	Turkey (roast, meat only,	
Grapefruit (half fruit)	15 calories	per 25g/1oz)	40 calories

in the body, requiring a great deal of energy. The energy we waste on coping with this excess is energy which is lost to other more vital functions. At the same time, the excess is not merely eliminated. It hangs around in the system as toxic waste, a condition whose detrimental effect on our health is accepted but not yet fully explored. What is beyond question is that it must be carried round as extra pounds.

In the last few years, nutritionists have begun to distinguish between two types of protein – animal and plant. We have always assumed that animal protein was *the* necessary kind for human health. But since all the animals we eat receive their protein from plants, it is becoming accepted that we can bypass our carnivore cravings and eliminate most, if not all, animal flesh from our diet without suffering undue harm. Even if you do *like* meat, poultry and fish and wish to keep them as a regular part of your diet, it would be wise to cut down appreciably on animal protein and up your vegetable quotient.

Salt

Sodium chloride is found naturally in many foods and is essential for a healthy body. But with the passage of time, particularly with the popularity of convenience and 'junk' foods, our consumption of salt – and our taste for it – has increased beyond what most experts consider healthy.

On average we consume about 12g a day; ordinary individuals need no more than 3–5g. If you live in a hot climate, work in a particularly physical job, or exercise regularly, you may require a little extra, though 12g is still more than anyone requires. Excess salt has been shown to be linked to high blood pressure and may also affect the efficient function of the kidneys. Certainly it does hamper waste elimination, bloating the body with retained water.

In order to cut down on salt intake, first remove salt containers from the table. Don't encourage the unthinking sprinkling of salt over food that many people indulge in. Next, try cutting salt out of most of your cooking. You will probably want to continue adding a pinch of salt to your cooking water for potatoes, pasta and rice, but make it as little as possible. Forego adding salt to vegetables as they cook, or to fish, meat or poultry. Experiment more with fresh herbs and spices – part of the modern passion for salt is little more than bored taste-buds! A simple dash of cayenne and pepper will add a quick, healthy fillip if salt still seems lacking. But you'll be surprised at how soon you will become accustomed to the 'real' taste of food without salt. Remember it's just that salt has become the MSG of the occidental table!

ELIMINATING THE WEED

Overeating can be an addiction, and smoking certainly is. The anti-smoking campaigns in the media in the last few years have made everyone aware of the risks we run if we continue to smoke. But knowing is not doing, and many people find it well nigh impossible to kick the habit. But lack of success in the past should not defeat you; if you are a smoker, stopping is probably the single most important step you can take toward better health and a longer life – even more important than losing weight.

If you are an overweight smoker, and you are determined to lose weight, both for your health and appearance, then before you begin a planned diet you should cut out smoking. Tobacco kills vitamins and lowers the body's resistance to disease, particularly to air-borne viruses – a side effect you should be aware of if you are cutting down on body-building food intake – and it also has a depressant effect on appetite. This last might seem to be an asset if you are trying to lose weight, but in actual fact it merely acts as a mask to the body's natural craving for food. If

A BAKER'S DOZEN TOP FIBRE FOODS

	Fibre content (per 100g unless stated)
Whole fibre bran	9.9g
Frozen peas	7.8g
Baked beans	7.3g
Wholewheat pasta	6.0g
Nuts	4.9g
Wholewheat flour	4.8g
Wholewheat flake cereal (per 30g serving)	3.8g
Baked potato with skin	3.4g
Muesli (per 40g serving)	3.0g
Wholewheat bread (per 30g slice)	2.6g
Dried fruit and nuts	2.5g
Fresh fruit (pear or apple) with skin	2.2g
Raw or crisp-cooked vegetables (cauliflower, broccoli, carrots, etc)	2.1g

(and hopefully when) you do finally quit, it may create more of a problem than if you gird your mental loins at the outset and make up your mind to do it first and foremost.

Most experts advise that if you have made up your mind to stop smoking, you will probably stand a better chance of being successful if you can go 'cold turkey' – in other words, stop smoking all at once. This may seem like an impossible demand to make on someone who has smoked 20–60 cigarettes a day, but psychologically it works better for most people than attempting the 'slowly does it' campaign of a cigarette less every day. But only you can decide the best way to quit – it's not the way, it's the quitting that counts!

LOSING WEIGHT AND KEEPING IT DOWN

If you are actively trying to lose weight, you should attempt to keep your daily intake down to 1,000–1,200 calories. Since an average-sized woman would be eating 2,000–2,300 calories a day to maintain her normal weight, the reduction should result in a loss of about 2lb a week. This gradual slimming – based on a sensible and varied diet, ideally accompanied by an hour of regular exercise two to three times a week – is far better for you than the more drastic 500–800 calorie regimes advocated by some diet gurus. It also makes more sense when it comes to keeping to your target weight once you have reached it. You will have educated your stomach – and your taste buds – to appreciate a whole spectrum of foods rich in low-fat protein, fibre and complex carbohydrates.

Finally, remember that keeping your weight at a healthy and attractive level will not always be a battle. Once you have established better eating habits, cut out the empty calorie foods, and achieved your target weight by a slow, careful process of calorie control, you should find staying there a natural follow-up. If you continue to eat the same kind of foods, and only increase your intake to the normal 2,000 mark by eating a little bit more of the same, life and the measuring tape should hold no terrors for you.

SLIM START BREAKFASTS

Breakfast has often tended to be an all-or-nothing affair. Traditionally, 'real men' like farmers and factory workers would fuel up with a 'hot breakfast' – eggs, toast, bacon or sausage (sometimes both!), grilled tomato and coffee – while many office workers rushed off to catch their train with no breakfast at all. Neither extreme really suits today's greater awareness of healthy living. Most men *and* women, whether at desk jobs or coping with demanding small children, should start the day with a light but nutritious breakfast – something low in fat and sugar but high in fibre and energy-giving carbohydrates. Just a slice of wholemeal toast lightly spread with honey or marmalade (if you *must* have 'butter', use a low-fat substitute) is ideal; but if you want to vary the way you start your days, the ideas below are inventive alternatives.

[One note of caution: Try to cut down on coffee. It has no calories of its own, but it does slow down the metabolic rate, making it harder to burn up the calories you do consume. You will be far better off with a 140ml (5fl oz) glass of unsweetened grapefruit or orange juice at only 50 calories, or a mug of hot water with a squeezed lemon quarter which has almost none. The latter has the additional positive property of speeding up your digestive juices.]

TANGY BANANA SQUASH
— 60 calories —

1 large banana, peeled and sliced
Juice of 1 large orange
Juice of 1 large lemon
225ml (8fl oz) low-fat yoghurt
Dash nutmeg

Put the sliced banana and the fruit juices into a blender or food processor bowl and whizz until smooth. With the motor running pour in the yoghurt and whizz until thoroughly combined and creamy. Serve each glass with a sprinkling of nutmeg. (The squash will keep covered in the refrigerator for 2–3 days.)

MAKES 3 SERVINGS

STUFFED GRAPEFRUIT
— 70 calories each —

1 grapefruit, halved, pith and flesh removed
2 stalks celery, finely chopped
50g (2oz) cottage cheese
2 carrots, grated
1 tsp fresh mint, finely chopped
1 tsp fresh chives, finely chopped
1 tsp pine nuts

Turn the grapefruit shells over so that they can drain. Place the separated grapefruit segments in a bowl, and add the celery, cottage cheese, grated carrots, mint and chives, and toss very gently to combine. Divide the stuffing between the two shells. Sprinkle each with the pine nuts. If not eating both grapefruit halves at the same time, keep the remaining filling in the bowl until ready to use.

MAKES 2 SERVINGS

LOW-CAL CHICKEN PÂTÉ TOAST
—— 140 calories ——

1 piece wholewheat toast
25g (1 oz) chicken pâté spread
1 small apple, thinly sliced

Spread the warm toast with the chicken pâté spread. Top with the apple slices.

SERVES 1

MUESLI YOGHURT
—— 145 calories ——

150g (6 oz) natural yoghurt
2 tbsp crunchy muesli
1 orange, divided into segments

Stir the yoghurt into the muesli in a bowl. Top with the orange segments.

SERVES 1

MEXICAN EGG
—— 150 calories ——

1 large egg
1 tbsp finely chopped red pepper
1 tbsp finely chopped green onion
1 tsp fresh chopped parsley
Pinch each cayenne, cumin, pepper and coriander seeds
1 piece wholewheat toast

Whisk all the ingredients except the toast together in a bowl. Divide the mixture between two non-stick cups of an egg poacher. Poach them, covered, until set. Turn out each cup onto a toast triangle.

SERVES 1

CHEESY FRUIT SCONES
—— 140 calories each ——

275g (10oz) wholewheat flour
4 tsp baking powder
Pinch salt
50g (2oz) butter
50g (2oz) low-fat cheese spread
275g (10oz) can crushed pineapple, drained
2 tbsp low-fat milk
1 large egg, beaten
Low-fat milk to glaze

In a bowl mix the flour, baking powder and salt together. Rub in the butter with the hands, then add the low-fat cheese spread and work in with the hands. Stir in the pineapple and the milk, break in the egg, and work to a dough. On a floured board, roll out the dough 1cm (½in) thick and cut out 12 6cm (2½in) rounds. Place on a greased baking tray, brush with the milk and bake in a preheated 200°C, 400°F, Gas 6 oven for 15 minutes until risen. Serve with low-calorie spread. (The scones will keep well in an air-tight container. Heat briefly before eating.)

MAKES 12 SCONES

SNEAKY OMELET
—— 140 calories ——

1 large egg
1 egg white
Pinch salt and pepper
1 tsp vegetable oil
1 tbsp chopped chives

With a fork, stir the egg and egg white together until blended, then stir in the seasoning. Pour the oil into a non-stick pan, turn it to coat, then pour in the egg and cook, lifting the edges. Sprinkle the chives over the omelet, allow to just set, then fold over and slide out onto a plate.

SERVES 1

ALMOST VEGETARIAN HOT LUNCHES

When you are trying to lose weight or to keep your weight down, it sometimes seems like needless fuss making a 'proper cooked lunch'. But there are times when nothing less will do – on a chilly winter's or rainy spring day, or when the family are at home, or on weekends when everyone welcomes a change from the routine of packed lunches and wine bar grub. The following recipes are quick to prepare and very low in calories. Rich in vegetables and complex carbohydrates, they fill you up and not out.

HEARTY FISH PIES

350 calories per serving

25g (1oz) butter
1 small onion, chopped
25g (1oz) plain flour
280ml (½pt) semi-skimmed milk
Salt and pepper
50g (2oz) Cheddar cheese, grated
Good pinch dry mustard
350g (12oz) cooked haddock or cod
350g (12oz) cooked mashed potato

Melt the butter in a frying pan and sauté the onion until soft, about 5 minutes. Sprinkle the flour over, stirring and cook for 1 minute. Gradually add the milk, stirring, and bring the mixture to the boil. As the sauce thickens add the seasoning, cheese and mustard to taste. Flake the fish and carefully stir it into the sauce. Spoon the mixture into four small dishes.

Place the potato in a piping bag fitted with a star nozzle. Starting from the centre, pipe in an outward spiral to cover the pies. Place under a low grill and cook until golden brown, about 10 minutes. (Since this is so filling, it needs only a small green salad to accompany it.)

(Pictured opposite)   SERVES 4

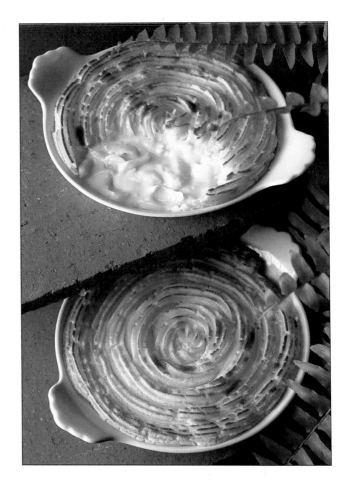

NUTTY CELERY AND RICE
260 calories per serving

8 stalks celery, trimmed and pared
175ml (6fl oz) chicken consommé
5 tbsp white wine
1½ tbsp chopped natural almonds
4 spring onions, finely chopped
1 tsp butter
Freshly ground pepper
100g (4oz) warm cooked brown rice

Slice the celery thinly and place in a 23cm (9in) baking dish. Pour the consommé and wine over, sprinkle with the almonds and spring onions and dot with the butter. Cover and bake in a preheated 200°C/400°F/Gas 8 oven for 15–20 minutes. Uncover, stir gently and then continue to cook for another 15 minutes, or until most of the liquid has evaporated, and you are left with a browned, thickened sauce. Season with pepper to taste. Divide the warm rice onto two plates and pour the celery mixture over them.

SERVES 2

TOMATO KEDGEREE
280 calories per serving

1 onion, peeled and chopped
1 tsp sunflower oil
100g (4oz) brown rice, cooked
350g (12oz) smoked haddock, cooked, skinned, boned and flaked
Salt and pepper
2 tbsp freshly chopped parsley
225g (8oz) tomatoes, sliced
2 hard-boiled eggs, shelled and sliced

Sauté the onion in the sunflower oil in a non-stick saucepan. Scrape it into a bowl and add the rice, smoked haddock, salt and pepper to taste, and parsley. Place one-third of the mixture in an ovenproof dish and cover with three quarters of the tomatoes. Top this with another layer of rice. Add a layer composed of the sliced eggs, then spread over the remaining rice. Use the remaining sliced tomatoes to make a decorative pattern. Cover the dish and bake in a preheated oven at 180°C/350°F/Gas 4 for 30 minutes. Serve immediately. (Any not used at once can be reheated or served cold.)

SERVES 4

CHEESY ORZO PRIMAVERA
260 calories per serving

280 ml (½pt) chicken stock or broth made from 1 cube and water
100g (4oz) orzo (small, rice-shaped pasta)
1½ tbsp unsalted butter
1 tbsp finely chopped shallots
1 large carrot, cut into small cubes
100g (4oz) green beans, diced
100g (4oz) frozen peas, thawed
1 courgette, diced
4 tbsp freshly grated Parmesan or Gruyère cheese
Freshly ground pepper
1 tbsp finely chopped spring onion

Bring the stock to boiling point in a saucepan and add the orzo. Reduce the heat to low, cover, and cook until the pasta is tender and the liquid almost absorbed. Remove from the heat and let rest.

Heat the butter in a frying pan over low heat. Stir in the shallots and cook for about 2 minutes, then add the carrots and beans and cook for a further 2 minutes. Stir in the peas and cover. Cook, shaking once or twice, for another 2 minutes. Finally add the courgette, cover, and cook for 2 more minutes. Uncover and stir to combine.

Stir 3 tbsp of the Parmesan or the Gruyère into the orzo and toss until combined. Scrape the orzo into the vegetables and toss lightly. Sprinkle with the spring onions and the remainder of the cheese. Serve immediately.

SERVES 3

INDIAN BEAN ROLLS
190 calories per serving

225g (8oz) rose cacao or pinto beans
1 clove garlic
1 bay leaf
Salt to taste
½ tsp cumin seeds
2 tbsp finely chopped coriander leaves
4 wholewheat chapatis
(made with chapati mix)
150ml (5oz) 1% fromage frais

Soak the beans for several hours or overnight in water. Then drain and cover with 900ml (1½pt) water. Bring to the boil and cook for 1 minute on high heat. Then cover and turn off the heat and allow to stand for 1 hour. Then bring to the boil again, adding the garlic and bay leaf. Simmer, covered, for about 1½ hours.

Remove the bay leaf. Using a potato masher, mash the beans to a paste in the remaining liquid. Continue until the result is lumpy-smooth. If the mash is beginning to look as if it might be too runny, cook gently to reduce. Stir in the salt to taste, cumin seeds and coriander leaves.

Make the chapatis according to directions and keep warm. Fill each chapati with a quarter of the filling and top with some of the fromage frais. Form each chapati into a roll. Serve, if desired, with a simple green salad. (If you are only using part of the bean mix at one time, the remainder will keep, covered, for 2–3 days in the refrigerator.)

SERVES 4

GREEN, WHITE AND RED CURRY
70 calories per serving

½ cauliflower, divided into florets and washed
225g (8oz) broccoli, divided into florets and washed
1 onion, peeled and chopped
1 clove garlic, crushed
2 tbsp olive oil
½ tsp chilli powder
½ tsp turmeric
½ tsp ground coriander
½ tsp garam masala
Salt and ground pepper
200g (7oz) tin chopped tomatoes

Cook the cauliflower and the broccoli in a large pan of boiling salted water for about 5 minutes or until just tender-crisp. Drain well. In a large saucepan soften the onion and garlic in the oil, and cook until just coloured. Stir in the spices and cook for another 1 minute. Add the tomatoes, cauliflower and broccoli. Stir for 5 minutes, until the vegetables are warmed through and coated with the sauce. Serve with warmed wholewheat rolls (125 calories each).

(Pictured below)   SERVES 2

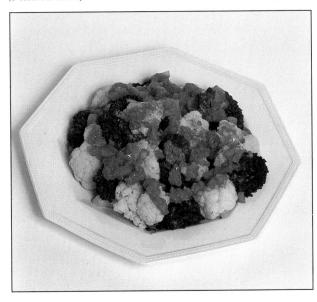

TURKISH STUFFED AUBERGINES
150 calories per serving

2 large aubergines
Salt and pepper
2 tbsp olive oil
2 large onions
225g (8oz) tomatoes
Large pinch cinnamon
¾ tsp brown sugar
1 clove garlic, minced
50g (2oz) raisins
1 tbsp pistachios
Finely chopped parsley

Trim the leaf ends from the aubergines and immerse them in a large saucepan. Pour boiling water over, cover and cook on a low boil for 10 minutes. Drain them, rinse in cold water and leave for 5 minutes. Cut in half lengthways, scoop out the flesh and reserve it. Arrange the shells on an oiled baking tray, season them and brush each shell lightly with a little oil – use no more than 1 tablespoon in all. Bake the aubergines in a pre-heated 180°C/350°F/Gas 4 oven for half an hour or until limp and lightly browned.

Meanwhile peel and chop the onions and tomatoes. Pour the remaining oil in a frying pan and sauté the onions for about 8 minutes or until golden. Then stir in the cinnamon, sugar, tomatoes, garlic and raisins. Cook for about 20 minutes, or until the mixture is thickened. Then stir in the chopped reserved aubergine flesh and the pistachios. Cook for a further 10–15 minutes.

Remove the aubergine shells from the oven, divide the mixture between them, and sprinkle the parsley over before serving. (If you do not use all the recipe at once, you can keep it in the fridge for a couple of days, or freeze it. It can then be served warm or cold.)

SERVES 4

GREEK VEGETABLE PIZZA
280 calories per serving

1 yeast pizza base mix
1 onion, peeled and chopped
2 tbsp olive oil
425g (15oz) can chopped tomatoes
Salt and ground pepper
4 tomatoes, thinly sliced
2 coloured peppers, seeded and sliced
12 stoned black olives
1 tsp dried oregano
1 clove garlic, chopped
50g (2oz) feta cheese, crumbled

Make the base according to instruction and roll out to a large circle. Place on a greased baking sheet.

Fry the onion in the oil until softened and just coloured. Add the chopped tomatoes and season with salt and pepper to taste. Remove from the heat and spread over the pizza base. Arrange the tomatoes, pepper rings and olives over the surface and sprinkle over the oregano and garlic. Bake at 200°C/400°F/Gas 6 for 30 minutes. Dot with pieces of feta halfway through the cooking.

(Pictured below)   SERVES 4

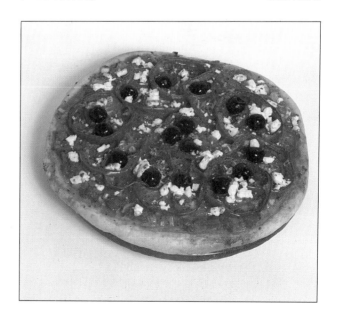

21

POTATO AND SPINACH BAKE
— 260 calories per serving —

2 medium potatoes, peeled and thinly sliced
375g (12oz) fresh spinach, washed trimmed and
chopped
Salt and pepper
½ tsp nutmeg
2 tbsp low-fat yoghurt
1 tbsp freshly grated Parmesan cheese

Put the potatoes in a saucepan and cover with water. Bring to the boil and cook until just tender. Drain and let them cool slightly.

Place the washed spinach in a saucepan with the water clinging to the leaves. Cook for about 15 minutes or until just wilted. Drain off excess water and mix in the seasoning, nutmeg and yoghurt. Place half the spinach in the bottom of a baking dish. Top with half the potatoes, arranged in a circle. Layer this with the remaining spinach and cover with the rest of the potatoes in a circular pattern. Salt and pepper the potatoes, brush them with the oil and sprinkle over the Parmesan. Bake in a preheated 200°C/400°F/Gas 6 oven for 15–20 minutes or until the potatoes are browned.

SERVES 2

HOT PRAWN-FILLED POTATO
— 155 calories —

Medium-sized jacket potato, scrubbed
25g (1oz) cottage cheese
25g (1oz) peeled prawns
2 drops Tabasco sauce
Pepper to taste
Freshly chopped chives

Prick the potatoes 3 or 4 times and oil the skin lightly with safflower or sunflower oil. Bake in a 200°C/400°F/Gas 6 oven for 1 hour or until soft.

In a bowl mix the cottage cheese, prawns and Tabasco sauce together. Cut open the top of the potato and squeeze the potato to force up the flesh. Pile in the filling, and top with a sprinkling of chopped chives. Serve immediately.

SERVES 1

SAUTÉED CHICKEN AND VEGETABLES WITH LEMON-ORANGE ZING
— 250 calories per serving —

Grated rind and segments of 1 small orange
1 clove garlic, minced
2 tbsp finely chopped fresh parsley
½ tsp fresh chopped tarragon
3 tbsp unsalted butter
1 shallot, thinly sliced
175g (6oz) baby French green beans
175g (6oz) baby oriental corn cobs
2 small courgettes, cut into matchsticks
½ each red, yellow and green pepper, cut into
matchsticks
225g (8oz) cooked chicken breast, cut into
matchsticks
100g (4oz) mushrooms, sliced
Juice of 1 lemon

Combine the orange rind, garlic, parsley and tarragon in a bowl. Reserve.

Heat the butter in a wok or a large frying pan over medium heat. Add the shallot, beans and oriental corn cobs and cook, stirring for about 3 minutes. Add the courgettes and peppers, and cook for a further 3 minutes. Finally stir in the chicken pieces and mushrooms and cook for another 4 minutes, until everything is hot but still crisp. Sprinkle the orange seasoning, lemon juice and orange segments over, toss and serve.

(Pictured opposite) SERVES 4

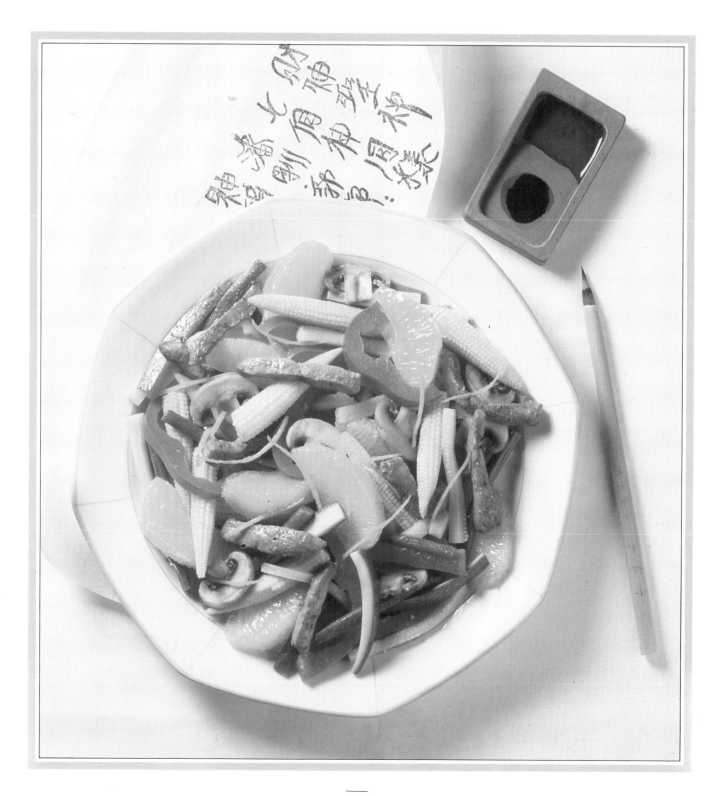

SALAD LUNCHES (for home, work and picnics)

Warm weather, a shortage of cooking time or simply inclination sometimes rule out a hot lunch at home. If you take your lunch to work, to munch at your desk or on a park bench, a hot meal is practically impossible, unless you have access to a kitchen. These are the times that a salad lunch comes into its own. It can be just as filling and comforting as a hot dish, while at the same time far lighter – a good thing if you are stuck behind a desk most of the day.

Picnics are the other time that salads are king. They are so versatile – ranging from the elegant to the honestly simple, from the highly spiced to the delicately flavoured. A salad certainly doesn't have to be made of lettuce; but it should be mainly composed of vegetables or greens dressed with a complimentary sauce. This latter is often where the calories creep in, so care should be taken to use low-fat ingredients as much as possible, and not to overdress the salad.

These are all main course salads. Serve only with an interesting bread (if it's interesting enough you won't miss the butter!), such as pitta, black bread, rye, pumpernickel, or whole wheat roll. This should add between 70–125 calories.

HEARTY GREEK SALAD
—— *340 calories* ——

1 small head Webb, Iceburg or Cos lettuce
½ each red and yellow peppers cut into strips
1 small onion, cut into slices
2 Mediterranean tomatoes, sliced
75g (3oz) feta cheese, cubed
10 black Greek olives

DRESSING
2 tbsp red wine
1 tbsp virgin olive oil
1 clove garlic, finely chopped
Dash sugar
pepper to taste

Make the dressing by combining all ingredients in order in a small bottle. Shake until fully emulsified.

Place the lettuce, peppers, onion, tomato, cheese and olives in a large salad bowl. Pour the dressing over and toss thoroughly. Serve immediately.

SERVES 2

TEXAN BEAN SALAD
—— *140 calories* ——

75g (3oz) kidney beans, soaked overnight
2 tsp olive oil
1 tbsp white wine vinegar
1 clove garlic
¼ tsp ground coriander
¼ tsp ground cumin
¼ tsp chilli powder
200g (7oz) cucumber, cut into chunks

Drain the beans and place them in a saucepan to cover with water. Bring to the boil and cook hard for 10 minutes, then lower the heat and cover. Cook for about 30 minutes or until the beans are tender.

Drain the beans. Blend the oil together with all the spices, pour over the beans, toss them, and leave to marinate until warm. Then add the cucumber, toss lightly, and chill. (This will keep for 2–3 days in the fridge.)

SERVES 2

Thai Chicken and Mango Salad

————— 275 calories per serving —————

6 tbsp fresh lime juice
2 tbsp fish sauce (nam pla) from oriental market
1cm (½in) ginger root, skinned and slivered
225g (8oz) whole chicken breast
½ head cos lettuce, shredded
Handful fresh mint leaves
Handful fresh coriander leaves
50g (2oz) bean sprouts
1 medium mango, peeled, stoned, and cubed
4 radishes, thinly sliced
1 small red onion, thinly sliced
1½ tbsp sunflower oil
Salt and pepper
Dash red pepper flakes
15g (½oz) peanuts

Combine half the lime juice, half the fish sauce and the ginger in a small bowl. Place the chicken into a glass or enamel dish and pour this marinade over it. Cover with cling film and let rest, turning occasionally, for 30 minutes.

Meanwhile, toss the lettuce, mint and coriander leaves, and bean sprouts together in a large bowl. Sprinkle the mango, radishes and red onion over the top. Make a dressing of the remaining lime juice and fish sauce, sunflower oil, and salt. Add pepper and the pepper flakes to taste. Whisk until emulsified. Reserve.

Heat a non-stick frying pan or wok over medium heat. Add the chicken breast and sauté, turning frequently, until it is cooked through. This will take about 10–12 minutes. Remove from the pan and let cool slightly. Then slice into thin strips. Add the strips to the salad. Just before serving, pour the dressing over the salad and toss well. Sprinkle with the peanuts and serve immediately.

Serves 2

Acapulco Fish Salad

————— 180 calories per serving —————

675g (1½lb) monkfish fillets
2 large tomatoes, cored and diced
65ml (2½fl oz) fresh lime juice
1 clove garlic, finely chopped
75g (3oz) pimento-stuffed olives, sliced
1 tbsp capers, drained
2 spring onions, thinly sliced
Small handful coriander, chopped
Lime wedges

Place the fish in a baking dish, with the fillets overlapping. Cover and bake in a preheated 200°C/400°F/Gas 6 oven, until just opaque in the thickest part, about 15 minutes. Let cool; cover and chill for at least 3 hours.

Lift out the fish, pull out and discard any stray bones. Break the fish into chunks. In a large bowl combine the tomatoes, lime juice, garlic, olives, capers, onions, coriander and fish; mix lightly. Season to taste. Allow to set for at least a short while before serving garnished with lime wedges. (It will keep for up to 2 days.)

Serves 4

CURRIED CHICKEN COUSCOUS SALAD

400 calories per serving

350g (12oz) boned and skinned chicken breasts
450ml (³⁄4pt) chicken broth
225g (8oz) couscous
35g (1¹⁄2oz) raisins
1 tbsp curry powder
½ tsp dried thyme
3 tbsp chopped fresh parsley
1 carrot, shredded
225g (8oz) can artichoke hearts, drained
1 red pepper, finely chopped
1 small red onion, chopped
4 lettuce leaves, washed and dried
8 cherry tomatoes, washed
1 medium cantaloupe, cut into wedges and seeded
1 lemon, cut into wedges

DRESSING
175ml (6fl oz) low-calorie yoghurt
1 tbsp honey

Put the chicken breast into the broth in a saucepan over high heat. Bring to the boil; cover and remove from heat. Let stand about 18 minutes, until the breasts are cooked through. Lift out the pieces and allow to cool.

Bring the broth to the boil again. Add the couscous, curry, raisins and thyme; stir and return to the boil; cover, remove from the heat and let stand until the couscous completely absorbs the liquid, about 10 minutes.

Meanwhile cut the chicken into thin strips. Stir the chicken, parsley, carrot, artichoke hearts, pepper and onion into the couscous. Cover and chill for at least 2 hours.

Make up the dressing. Stir in the yoghurt and honey together in a bowl until they are thoroughly combined. To serve, place a lettuce leaf on each plate, spoon some of the mixture onto it. Arrange the tomatoes and melon wedges decoratively on the couscous and accompany with a lemon wedge. Pour a little dressing over each serving. (If all the salad is not used at once, keep refrigerated for up to 2 days with the lettuce, tomato and melon, as well as the dressing, separate.)

SERVES 4

AVOCADO, GRAPEFRUIT AND PRAWN SALAD

235 calories per serving

2 grapefruit
2 avocados
225g (8oz) cooked prawns
1 fresh lime
Watercress to decorate

Follow this easy way to peel the grapefruit: place the fruit in a bowl and pour over boiling water to cover. Leave for 2 minutes, then remove and allow to cool. Cut a slice from the top of each fruit, then cut the peel and pith off in vertical strips to reveal the flesh. Use a very sharp small knife. After all the peel and pith have been removed, cut in between the membranes of each segment and separate them.

Peel the avocados, cut them in half lengthways and remove the stones. Cut the flesh into thin slices. Place a slice of avocado over each slice of grapefruit and arrange attractively in lines down a serving plate. Add the cooked prawns in decorative lines. Garnish with watercress leaves. Cut the lime and squeeze the juice over before serving.

SERVES 4

PECAN-ORANGE SALAD

170 calories per serving

4 oranges
50g (2oz) shelled pecan halves
½ head curly endive, washed and drained
100g (4oz) Webb lettuce or watercress

DRESSING
3 tbsp fresh lemon juice
4 tbsp sunflower oil
1 clove garlic, peeled and crushed
1 tsp finely grated orange rind
1 tbsp finely chopped parsley
Salt and ground pepper

Finely grate 1 teaspoon orange rind from an orange and reserve. With a sharp knife, cut the top and bottom off the oranges. Remove the rind and the pith. Carefully cut each segment out of the oranges over the serving bowl to catch the juice. Pip the segments, then toss them with the nuts, endive and lettuce. Pour the dressing ingredients into a screw-top jar and shake well. Just before serving pour over the salad. (This salad will not keep for any length of time.)

(Pictured below)   SERVES 4

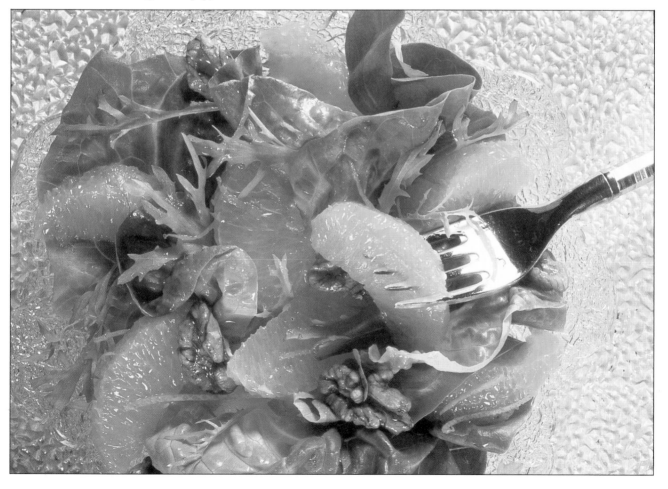

WINTER VEGETABLE SALAD
120 calories per serving

225g (8oz) red cabbage, shredded
100g (4oz) carrots, peeled and grated
1 onion, skinned and grated
100g (4oz) Brussels sprouts, shredded
1 large crisp red apple, diced
2 tbsp lemon juice

DRESSING
140ml (5fl oz) carton low-fat yoghurt
1 tsp grated orange rind
½ tsp caraway seeds
Large pinch nutmeg
Salt and pepper

You can use the grating blade of a food processor to shred and grate the vegetables, if you wish. Mix all the salad ingredients in a large bowl and moisten with the lemon juice to prevent discolouration. Whisk the dressing ingredients together and pour over the salad immediately before serving. (If you are not eating all of the salad at once, do not dress the reserved vegetables until used. They, and the mixed dressing, will keep, covered securely and chilled, for 2 days.)

SERVES 2

SALAD NIÇOISE
395 calories per serving

225g (8oz) new potatoes, scrubbed, boiled until tender and sliced
200g (7oz) can tuna in brine, drained
100g (4oz) green beans, trimmed and cooked until tender-crisp
Lettuce leaves
A few slices of cucumber
Four anchovy fillets, cut lengthways
6 cherry tomatoes
12 black olives

DRESSING
60ml (2fl oz) chicken broth
1 tbsp olive oil
2 tbsp wine vinegar
2 tsp Dijon mustard
1 clove garlic, crushed
Salt and pepper

Make the dressing by whisking all ingredients together in a small bowl. Taste and adjust the seasoning.

Place the potato slices in a bowl. Flake the tuna and add most of it to the bowl, together with the beans. Arrange the lettuce leaves and slices of cucumber on a a serving platter. Pour just enough of the dressing over the tuna mixture to moisten well. Pile the mixture onto the platter. Sprinkle over the remaining tuna flakes, criss-cross the anchovy fillets on top and garnish the platter with the olives and tomatoes. Serve immediately. (If taking on a picnic, dress the salad just before serving.)

SERVES 2

SMOKED MACKEREL AND APPLE SALAD

290 calories per serving

350g (12oz) 'hot smoked' mackerel fillets
1 large dessert apple, cored and chopped
2 stalks celery, chopped
25g (1oz) raisins
Salt and ground black pepper
1 tsp fresh lemon juice

DRESSING
3 tbsp natural yoghurt
2 tbsp mayonnaise

Cut the mackerel fillets into cubes and place them in a large bowl. Mix in the apple, celery, raisins, seasoning and lemon juice. Mix mayonnaise and yoghurt together and pour over the salad, stir carefully until coated. Serve on a bed of crisp lettuce, if desired. (If all the salad is not used immediately, it may be kept refrigerated – without the shredded lettuce – for up to 2 days.)

(Pictured below)   SERVES 4

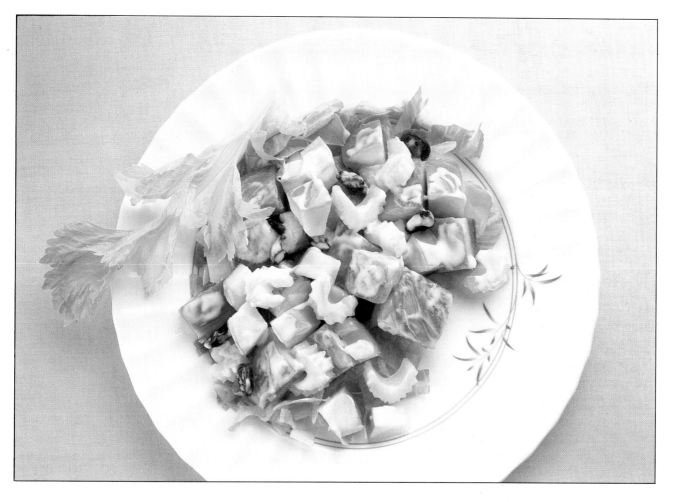

SOUP, SANDWICHES AND SNACKS

Snacking during the day is always a hazard to a healthy diet, especially if you are trying to lose weight. On the other hand, there are times when a snack is needed. When you are running late and have missed lunch, or have experienced a particularly taxing or energetic day, a little something, as Pooh said, is in order. Warming, vegetable-rich soup, a light wholesome sandwich, or a low-calorie piece of fruit can plug all holes and revive the system and your flagging spirits.

The dishes below are filling and delicious, while at the same time 'good for you' – far better than a chocolate bar or sweet biscuits. Keep the soups frozen and heat up when needed.

SPICY CARROT AND ORANGE SOUP
— 85 calories per serving —

25g (1oz) butter or margarine
450g (1lb) carrots, peeled and chopped
1 medium onion, peeled and chopped
1 clove garlic, finely chopped
2.5cm (1in) piece root ginger, peeled and sliced
560ml (1pt) chicken stock
2 oranges
Large pinch basil
Freshly ground black pepper
140ml (¼pt) Greek-style yoghurt
1 egg yolk

Melt the butter or margarine in a saucepan and add the carrots and onions. Cook the vegetables for about 5 minutes, then add the garlic, ginger and stock. Grate the rind from ½ an orange and squeeze the juice from both oranges. Add this to the soup and bring it to the boil. Turn down the heat and simmer, covered, for 15 minutes. When the carrots are tender, allow the soup to cool slightly, then purée it in batches in a blender or food processor. When smooth, add the basil and pepper to taste. Pour back into the saucepan and reheat gently. Take off the heat and whisk in the yoghurt and the egg yolk. Serve immediately. (The soup cannot be reheated once the yoghurt and egg yolk have been added; if the soup is to be frozen or refrigerated before use, do not add the yoghurt and egg yolk until just before serving.)

SERVES 4

LOW-CAL QUICKIE SNACKS	
I large apple	70 calories
Grapes (per grape)	5 calories
I medium orange	60 calories
I medium tangerine	35 calories
I carrot	30 calories
I medium tomato	25 calories
I slice wholewheat toast with low-calorie jam	95 calories
100g (4oz) plain low-calorie yoghurt	70 calories
I small hard-boiled egg	80 calories
2 fig biscuits	100 calories
I frozen juice bar	70–90 calories

TOMATO-RICE SOUP
120 calories per serving

25g (1oz) butter
1 onion, chopped
450g (1lb) ripe tomatoes, peeled, seeded and chopped
Salt and pepper
50g (2oz) long-grain rice
1.2l (2pt) chicken or vegetable stock
Pinch thyme
Bay leaf

Melt the butter in a heavy-based saucepan and cook the onion in it until lightly coloured, about 5–8 minutes. Add the tomatoes, and stir in the salt and pepper. Pour in the rice and the stock, add the thyme and bay leaf. Stir to combine and bring to the boil. Reduce the heat, cover and cook gently for 20 minutes, until the rice is soft. Remove the bay leaf and serve in warmed bowls. (This soup will keep, chilled, for 2–3 days.)

SERVES 4

ORIENTAL SPINACH AND PEPPER SOUP
50 calories per serving

450ml (¾pt) chicken stock
2 tbsp dry white wine
2 thin slices fresh ginger, skinned
100g (4oz) spinach leaves, washed and shredded
½ sweet red pepper, finely chopped
2 thin slices lime, chopped
¼ tsp cayenne pepper

Pour the stock, wine and ginger into a saucepan. Bring to the boil, then reduce the heat and simmer, uncovered, for about 5 minutes. Remove from the heat. Discard the ginger and stir in the spinach, red pepper, lime and cayenne. Serve at once.

SERVES 2

TANGY MUSHROOM SOUP
90 calories per serving

175g (6oz) mushrooms, washed and dried
50g (2oz) onion, thinly sliced
50g (2oz) carrots, peeled and sliced
1 tbsp butter
450ml (¾pt) chicken stock
Salt and pepper
Large pinch nutmeg
1 tsp Dijon mustard
1 tsp lemon juice
Dash Tabasco sauce
1 tbsp single cream or top of the milk

Leave a few mushrooms aside for garnish and slice the remainder. Toss the onion and carrots in with the butter into a non-stick saucepan and toss briefly until glazed, then cover and sweat for about 3 minutes. Uncover, stir in the sliced mushrooms, and cook, stirring, for a further 5 minutes. Pour in the stock, seasoning, spice and mustard, lemon juice and Tabasco. Bring to the boil, stirring, cover, and cook on low heat for half an hour. Remove from the heat and allow to cool slightly.

Purée the soup in a blender or food processor. If you wish it a little thinner, add water. Coarsely chop the reserved mushrooms, add to the soup, and reheat, just before serving stir in the cream. (Simply double the quantities for 4; the soup will keep in a refrigerator for 2–3 days. Add the cream just before serving.)

SERVES 2

GOURMET LOW-CALORIE OPEN SANDWICHES

Rye bread, thinly spread with low-calorie cream cheese mixed with chopped fruit chutney. Top with 2 thin slices smoked ham, watercress, and grinding of black pepper

190 calories

Raisin or currant bread, spread with a mixture of low-calorie cream cheese, raisins, dried apricots and cinnamon

160 calories

Wholewheat bread, spread with applesauce and topped with slice of gruyère and slice of pressed turkey breast

200 calories

Small pitta pocket stuffed with a mixture of chopped lettuce, 25g (1oz) feta, 1 medium chopped tomato and 50g (2oz) chopped cucumber, tossed in 1 tablespoon low-calorie yoghurt

195 calories

Rye bread, topped with 1 mashed sardine, 1 sliced hard-boiled egg, and 2 chopped spring onions

220 calories

Pumpernickel bread, spread with 25g (1oz) camembert, ½ sliced pear, and 5 walnut halves

290 calories

½ Italian roll, topped with 25g (1oz) sliced and mashed mozzarella, 1 medium sliced tomato, oregano, black pepper and ½ teaspoon olive oil drizzled over

220 calories

THICK LENTIL SOUP
95 calories per serving

1 large onion, peeled and chopped
4 stalks celery, chopped with leaves
2 large carrots, peeled and chopped
1 large parsnip, peeled and chopped
75g (3oz) split yellow lentils
2 tbsp chopped fresh parsley
900ml (1½pt) chicken stock
Salt and pepper

Place all the ingredients, saving a little of the parsley for garnish, and two-thirds of the stock, into a large saucepan. Bring to the boil, then lower the heat and simmer gently for about 1½ hours. Liquidise or sieve half the soup and return it to the pot with the remainder. This gives a soup with a lumpy, peasanty texture. Add the remainder of the stock and reheat, stirring. Stir in the chopped parsley before serving. (This soup freezes well and can be used a little at a time, if desired.)

(Pictured opposite)   SERVES 6

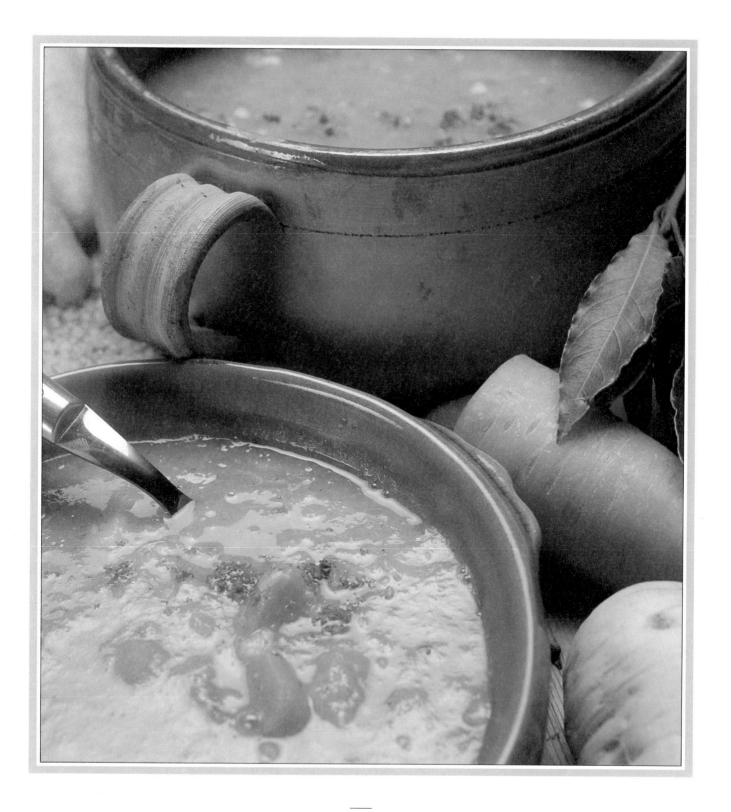

HEALTHY DINNERS

Dinner is probably the meal that causes the most problems to the dieter. It's hard enough denying yourself or 'being healthy' at lunchtime, but at least there are certain curbs automatically posed by time and custom. Unlike Mediterranean countries, we do not have hours off for lunch, nor are we in the habit of large family lunchtime gatherings in the middle of the week. We know that we still have several hours of concentrated work ahead and another meal to look forward to at the end of the working day. So all of these considerations operate to make us take our lunchtimes fairly carefully.

The same is not true of dinner. Work is over; you're back at home with your comfy clothes on. You feel you've earned that glass of wine, and the chance to let your hair down with friends, husband, lover or family over a good meal. If you're the one who's stayed at home all day, tackling the house and looking after the kids, you'll want to celebrate the homecoming of everyone else and the chance the talk over the day's happenings. In either case, a good meal helps to relax the body and spirit and wind up the day. Who wants to count calories and munch on a piece of dry toast at such a time?

The secret to keeping the weight down and energy up is to serve meals that are calorie intensive. Concentrate on foods where the calories are fibre-, protein- and complex carbohydrate-rich, so that you really feel satisfied. And design your dinner so that everyone can eat the same thing and enjoy it – with the recipes below, even the greediest red meat-and-potatoes man will feel he's had his fill!

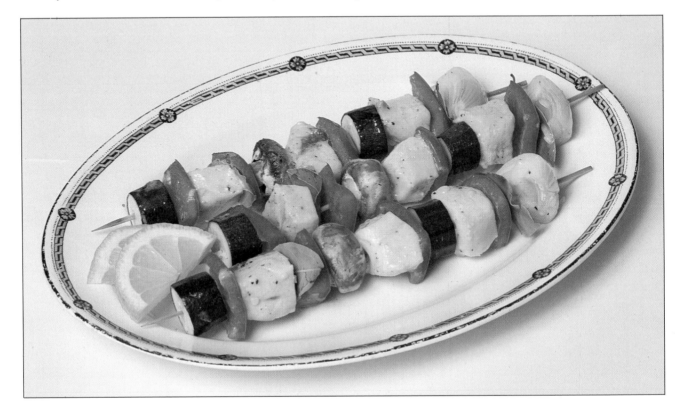

SWORDFISH KEBABS
265 calories per serving

6 tbsp soy sauce
2 tbsp dry sherry
2 tbsp sesame oil
1 spring onion, finely chopped
2 cloves garlic, crushed
1 tbsp peeled and chopped fresh ginger
Freshly ground pepper
675g (1½lb) swordfish steaks, cubed
100g (4oz) butter, softened
Fresh coriander, finely chopped
1½ tbsp wasabi paste (Japanese mustard-horseradish)
2 green or red peppers, cubed
2 small courgettes, cut into 3cm (1½in) pieces
4 bay leaves

Combine the soy sauce, sherry, oil, onion, garlic, ginger and pepper in a large bowl. Add the cubed swordfish and toss to coat. Refrigerate, covered, and marinate for 12–24 hours.

Make a paste of the softened butter, fresh coriander and wasabi paste. Reserve and allow to chill. Remove the fish from the marinade and thread pieces alternately with the pepper cubes and courgette pieces onto 4 long skewers. Interspace with pieces of the bay leaves. Preheat the grill and cook the kebabs for about 6–8 minutes, or until done. Turn once or twice. Serve with wasabi butter; allow 1 tablespoon per kebab.

(pictured opposite)   SERVES 4

GRATIN OF SPRING GREENS
300 calories per serving

50g (2oz) dry breadcrumbs
8 large cloves garlic, peeled
175g (6fl oz) Greek-style yoghurt
120ml (4fl oz) milk
Salt and pepper
675g (1½lb) spring greens, rinsed and chopped
3 tbsp olive oil
2 shallots, chopped
4 large eggs
100g (4oz) grated Gruyère cheese
Large pinch nutmeg
2 tbsp grated Parmesan cheese

Preheat the oven to 180°C/350°F/Gas 4. Grease a large baking dish, coat with the breadcrumbs and shake out the excess. Place 6 cloves of garlic in a small saucepan, cover with water and bring to the boil. Reduce heat and simmer until the garlic is tender, about 15 minutes. Drain the garlic and add to a blender or food processor, along with the yoghurt and milk. Blend until smooth; season to taste and reserve.

Bring a large saucepan of water to the boil. Add the spring greens, cover and cook until just wilted, about 2 minutes. Drain the greens, squeeze dry and shred finely. Heat the oil over medium heat. Mince the remaining garlic, add to the oil with the shallots and sauté until soft – do not allow to brown. Stir in the spring greens and cook a further 2 to 3 minutes.

In a large bowl whisk together the eggs, garlic cream and Gruyère. Stir in the greens mixture and combine thoroughly. Spoon into the prepared baking dish, season with the nutmeg and then sprinkle over the Parmesan. Place the dish in a large baking pan and pour boiling water in the pan to come halfway up the sides of the dish. Bake in the oven for about 35 minutes, or until the pudding is puffed, golden and a cocktail stick inserted comes out clean. Let cool slightly before serving. (Serve with baked or boiled potatoes or corn on the cob.)

SERVES 6

RED PEPPER COD
— 120 calories per serving —

450g (1lb) cod fillet, in 4 pieces
Salt and ground pepper
Large pinch nutmeg
1 small onion, chopped
Rind of ½ lemon, grated
1 small red pepper, seeded and shredded
150ml (5fl oz) yoghurt
2 tsp tomato ketchup
1 tsp tomato paste
Large dash Worcester sauce

Season the fillets with the salt, pepper and nutmeg. Spread the chopped onion and grated lemon over the base of a baking dish. Lay the fillets on top.

In a bowl, combine the red pepper, yoghurt, ketchup, tomato paste and Worcester sauce. Season with salt and pepper to taste. Pour the sauce over the fish, cover with aluminium foil and cook in a preheated 200°C/400°F/Gas 6 oven for about 20 minutes, or until the cod is tender. (Serve with brown rice – about 50g (2oz) uncooked weight per person.)

SERVES 4

MONKFISH PROVENÇAL
— 135 calories per serving —

1 tsp sunflower oil
1 clove garlic, crushed
1 large onion, chopped
175g (6oz) mushrooms, sliced
1 small red pepper, deseeded and sliced
1 small green pepper, deseeded and sliced
2 small courgettes, sliced
175g (6oz) canned chopped tomatoes
450g (1lb) monkfish fillets, cubed
Salt and ground pepper
6 black olives
Watercress to garnish

Heat the oil in a non-stick pan and sauté the garlic, onion, mushrooms, peppers and courgettes. Add the tomatoes, cover, and simmer for 2 minutes. Uncover and cook on high for about 5 minutes, until the liquid is reduced. Stir in the monkfish cubes and simmer for another 5 minutes or until fish is just done. Adjust the seasoning and serve garnished with the olives and watercress. (Accompany with 50g/2oz each uncooked weight of wholewheat pasta, an additional 200 calories.)

SERVES 4

SPINACH LASAGNE
— 300 calories per serving —

1 large onion, grated
200g (7oz) cooked spinach, fresh or defrosted
225g (8oz) ricotta or cottage cheese
Salt and ground pepper
Large pinch cayenne
3 tbsp low-fat spread
4 tbsp plain flour
450ml (¾pt) skimmed milk
Large pinch mustard powder
100g (4oz) easy cook lasagne
3 tbsp grated Parmesan cheese

Combine the onion, spinach, cheese, salt and pepper and cayenne in a bowl. Gently melt the low-fat spread in a saucepan and add the flour. Stir for about 1 minute, then gradually stir in the milk. Bring to the boil, stirring, until thickened. Simmer while adding the mustard and a little pepper. Spread a third of the bechamel over the bottom of a baking dish. Layer over half the lasagne. Top with half of the spinach and cheese mixture. Repeat the layers and top with a final layer of bechamel. Sprinkle the Parmesan on top. Bake in a preheated 200°C/400°F/Gas 6 oven for 45 minutes, or until browned and bubbling on top. (This only needs a tossed green salad.)

SERVES 4

CHICKEN AND PULSE CASSEROLE
450 calories per serving

75g (3oz) dried haricot beans
75g (3oz) dried kidney beans
4 chicken joints
2 tbsp cooking oil
2 large onions, chopped
4 tomatoes, chopped
100g (4oz) mushrooms, wiped and sliced
Salt and ground pepper

Soak the haricot and kidney beans overnight in water. Drain. Place the beans in a casserole with water to cover, bring to the boil and then simmer for about 1 hour. Strain the beans, reserving 300ml (½ pint) of the cooking liquid.

In a large flameproof casserole, fry the chicken joints in the oil until golden brown. Place the onions, tomatoes and mushrooms in the casserole, season well, and add the beans with the reserved liquor. Cover and cook in the centre of a preheated 180°C/350°F/Gas 4 oven for 1½ hours, or until the chicken is tender. (This casserole freezes well, if all is not needed at once.)

(Pictured below)   SERVES 4

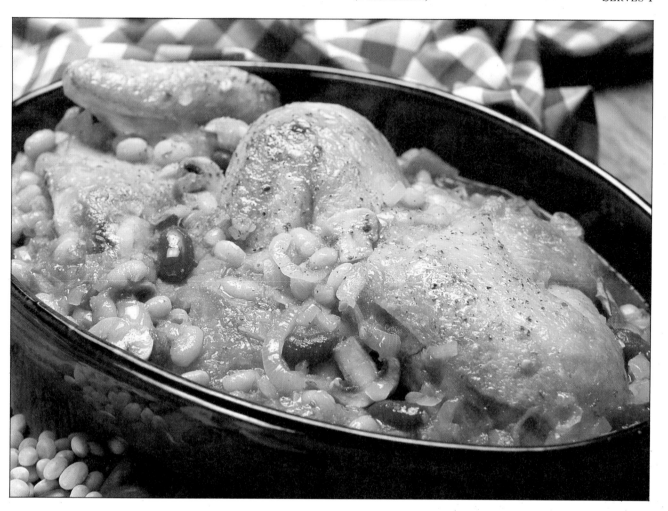

ITALIAN CHICKEN BREASTS

180 calories per serving

3 large chicken breasts, skinned, boned and halved
Flour
Salt and ground pepper
2 tbsp olive oil
120ml (4fl oz) white wine
120ml (4fl oz) chicken stock
12 fresh sage leaves
Large dash cayenne
2 small branches fresh rosemary

Dip the chicken pieces in the flour seasoned with salt and pepper. Pour the oil into a frying pan and heat; add the chicken pieces and sauté until golden on both sides. When the chicken is browned, drain off the oil and pour in the wine and stock. Turn the chicken in the sauce to coat and bring to bubbling. Cover each piece with two sage leaves, sprinkle with cayenne and shred the rosemary over. Cover and simmer the chicken for 15–20 minutes, until tender.

Remove the chicken to a serving dish. Increase the heat and reduce the liquid until it will just coat the chicken. Spoon the sauce over the breasts. (Serve on top of small helpings of potatoes mashed with low-fat spread and low-fat yoghurt.)

SERVES 6

PRAWN AND COTTAGE CHEESE SOUFFLÉ

300 calories per serving

1 tbsp butter or margarine
1½ tsp plain flour
140ml (¼pt) milk
Salt and ground pepper
2 eggs, separated
50g (2oz) cottage cheese with chives
225g (8oz) peeled prawns, fresh or defrosted
1 tbsp chopped fresh parsley

Preheat the oven to 180°C/350°F/Gas 4. Melt the butter in a saucepan, stir in the flour and cook for 1 minute. Remove from the heat and gradually stir in the milk. Return to a gentle heat and stir until the sauce thickens. Season to taste. Take off the heat again, and beat in the egg yolks. Stir in the cottage cheese and the prawns, reserving a few for decoration.

In a bowl, whisk the egg whites until stiff, and fold into the cottage cheese mixture, together with most of the parsley. Pour into a greased soufflé dish; sprinkle over the reserved prawns. Bake in the oven until risen and golden brown, about 30–35 minutes. Decorate with a sprinkling of parsley and serve immediately. (This goes particularly well with a green vegetable, such as broccoli or spinach.)
(Pictured below)

SERVES 2

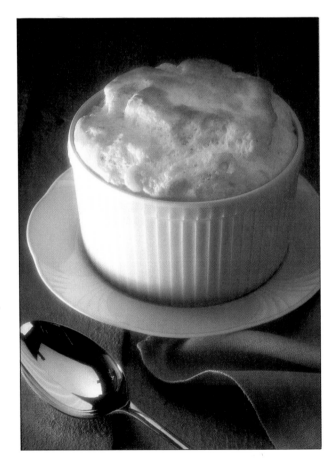

BRAISED STUFFED LETTUCE
250 calories per serving

200g (7oz) can black-eyed beans, drained
2 tbsp raisins
4 spring onions, chopped
225g (8oz) ricotta cheese
Salt and pepper
1 tsp cumin seed
½ tsp dill seeds
1 egg, beaten
1 iceberg lettuce
140ml (¼pt) basic chicken or vegetable stock
25g (1oz) butter
50g (2oz) Cheddar cheese, grated
25g (1oz) breadcrumbs
Paprika

Place the beans in a mixing bowl. Add the raisins, spring onions, ricotta cheese, salt and pepper to taste and the cumin and dill. Combine thoroughly, mashing the beans. Stir in the beaten egg.

Cut the lettuce into 4 wedges. Core the wedges and remove some of the smaller inner leaves. Stuff each of the wedges with some of the bean and cheese mixture and place in a baking dish. Pour over the basic stock, dot with butter, and bake, covered with foil, for about 30 minutes at 200°C/400°F/Gas 6. Uncover, sprinkle the wedges with the grated cheese, breadcrumbs and paprika and grill for about 5 minutes, or until brown and bubbling. (Serve with brown rice to mop up the juices.)

SERVES 4

TANDOORI CHICKEN
220 calories per serving

450ml (16fl oz) low-fat yoghurt
2 cloves garlic, crushed
2 tbsp fresh lime juice
1 tsp minced fresh ginger
½ tsp ground coriander
Pinch anise seeds
½ tsp chilli powder
½ tsp garam masala
Salt
2 pieces chicken, skinned

SAUCE
225ml (8fl oz) low-fat yoghurt
1 small cucumber, diced
1 medium carrot, finely chopped
Salt and pepper

Mix the ingredients for the tandoori marinade: the yoghurt, garlic, lime juice, ginger, coriander, anise, chilli powder, garam masala and salt to taste. Cut slits in the chicken pieces and add to the marinade, turning to coat. Leave to marinate for 6 hours or overnight.

Make the sauce by mixing together all the ingredients. Chill.

Preheat the oven to 180°C/350°F/Gas 4. Remove the chicken pieces from the marinade and place on a rack over baking dish. Cook for 30–40 minutes; serve immediately with the sauce and additional lime wedges.

SERVES 4

TOMATO HERRING
286 calories per serving

1 tsp sunflower oil
½ onion, sliced
4 herring, filleted
200g (7oz) can chopped tomatoes
1 tbsp lemon juice
1 tsp basil
½ tsp sugar
Salt and pepper

Heat the oil in a large shallow pan and cook the onion until soft and transparent. Add the herring fillets and cook for 2 minutes on both sides over a gentle heat. Add the tomatoes, lemon juice, basil, sugar and seasoning to taste. Cover and cook for a further 4 minutes. (Serve with plenty of Greek or pitta bread to mop up the sauces and a green salad.)
(Pictured right)   SERVES 4

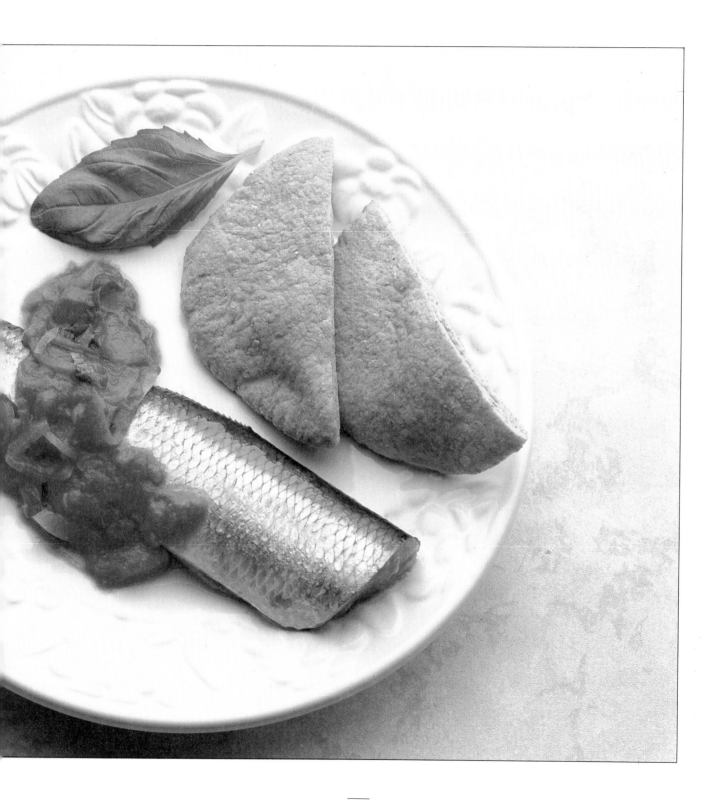

ENTERTAINING *(firsts and seconds)*

It's hard enough keeping the weight down when you're on your own or just with the family. Temptation still beckons – even when it's just you and the fridge door! But how much harder it is when the social calendar is full. Suddenly you are faced with desserts, unaccustomed first courses, and main courses swimming in cream and butter. If you are the guest, then you can take refuge in the thought that once in a while you need a break, and you can always make it up tomorrow by being particularly good. (Thank heavens calories are cumulative, and the damage done one day can be countermanded by the next. It's not like an exam!)

On the other hand, if you are the hostess, you may feel under a certain duress – especially if you entertain often. Somehow it doesn't seem right to count your calories during the week and then suddenly explode into an orgy of indiscriminate gorging when guests come and you are supposed to be the one in control. It may be difficult to keep three courses within the limits, especially if you are eating another meal during the day, but you can certainly try! The following recipes are all very low-calorie while at the same time festive – your guests will never know that they are 'being good' thanks to your careful planning – unless you tell them! You can choose a complimentary dessert from the next chapter.

FIRSTS

SCANDINAVIAN SALAD
—— *225 calories per portion* ——

100g (4oz) dried apple rings
350g (12oz) rollmop herrings
140ml (¼pt) low-fat yoghurt
1 tsp dill
Freshly ground pepper
Dill sprigs

Soak the apple rings in water for about 1 hour. Drain the rollmops and slice them into 1cm (½in) pieces. In a large bowl mix together the yoghurt, dill and pepper. Add the rollmops and the drained apple rings and toss lightly. Decorate with dill sprigs and serve with light caraway rye bread, if desired (approximately an extra 70 calories per small slice).

(Pictured opposite) SERVES 4

SCALLOP SEVICHE
—— *190 calories a serving* ——

900g (2lb) fresh scallops, halved
175ml (6fl oz) fresh lemon juice
175ml (6fl oz) fresh lime juice
1 purple onion, skinned and sliced
1 yellow pepper, thinly sliced
150g (5oz) stuffed green olives, sliced
2 tbsp olive oil
1 tbsp chopped fresh coriander
Rind of ½ lime, finely chopped
Salt
3 dashes Tabasco or hot pepper sauce

Combine all the ingredients in a large glass, earthenware or enamel bowl. Cover with cling film and refrigerate overnight. Just before serving, divide the seviche between 8 attractive glass dishes or bowls. Serve with thin slices of dark or black bread.

SERVES 8

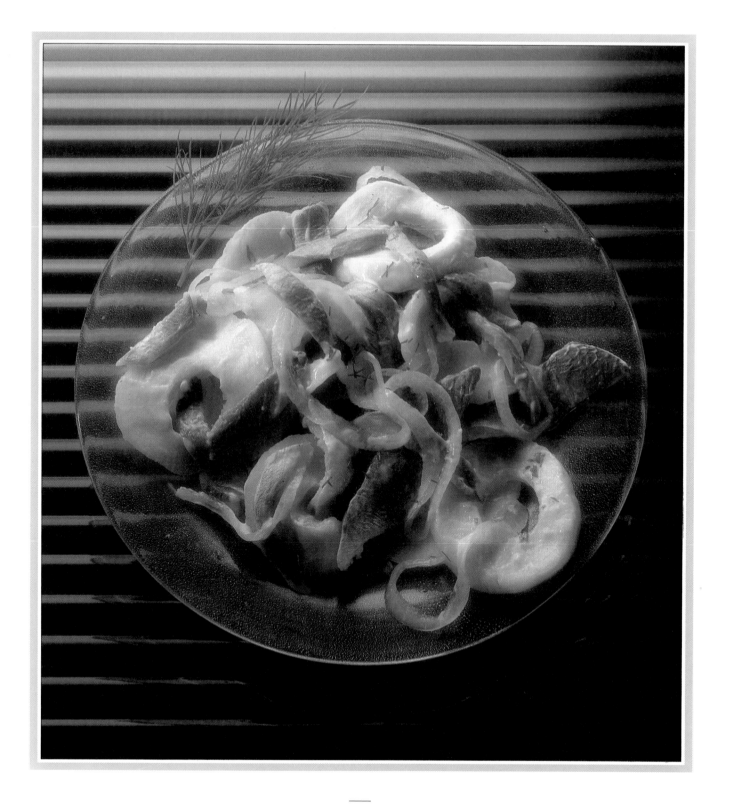

MARKET PÂTÉ

190 calories per serving
with toast

50g (2oz) butter
1 onion, peeled and chopped
2 cloves garlic, crushed
225g (8oz) button mushrooms, chopped
225g (8oz) large flat mushrooms, chopped
1 tbsp parsley, finely chopped
15g (½oz) walnuts, finely chopped
Salt and ground pepper
2 tbsp dry sherry
Chopped parsley for decoration
12 slices of wholewheat toast, cut into triangles

Melt the butter and cook the onion and the garlic until soft. Add the two types of mushroom, sauté gently to soften, then turn the heat up and cook until all the liquid evaporates. Scrape the mushrooms into the bowl of a food processor with the metal blade; add the parsley, walnuts, seasoning to taste and sherry. Process until roughly smooth. Decorate with the chopped parsley and serve with four triangles (2 pieces of toast) to each guest.
(Pictured below)   SERVES 6

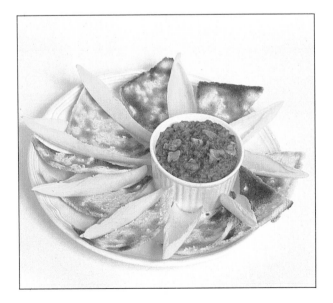

ARTICHOKES WITH VINAIGRETTE

140 calories per serving

6 artichokes, stem and leaves trimmed
1 lemon, cut into quarters
1 clove garlic, crushed
1 small onion, quartered
1 bay leaf

VINAIGRETTE
200ml (7fl oz) olive oil
90ml (3fl oz) sherry vinegar
1½ tsp chopped fresh oregano
1 clove garlic, crushed
Salt and pepper
1 tsp Dijon mustard

Plunge the artichokes into a large saucepan of cold water to cover halfway, then add the remaining cooking ingredients, with the salt to taste. Bring to the boil, then cover and reduce to simmer and cook until tender, 30–40 minutes. Remove the artichokes, drain thoroughly and allow to cool.

Meanwhile make the vinaigrette by whisking all the ingredients together in a small bowl. Pour a little of the vinaigrette in each of six ramekins and serve with the cooled artichokes on a large plate.
                                                    SERVES 6

CRUDITÉS AND CURRIED DIP
80 calories per serving

225ml (8fl oz) low-fat yoghurt
4 tbsp finely chopped spring onion
1 tsp curry paste
1 green pepper, cut into strips
8–12 radishes
1 small cauliflower, cut into florets
4 large celery stalks, cut into matchsticks
4 medium carrots, cut into matchsticks

Mix together the yoghurt, spring onion and curry paste and spoon into an attractive bowl. Arrange all the cut vegetables around the bowl on a large platter. Serve.

(Pictured below)   SERVES 4

STUFFED MUSHROOMS
180 calories per serving

8 large flat field mushrooms
225g (8oz) white crab meat
50g (2oz) low-fat soft cheese
Salt and ground pepper
1 tbsp chopped chives
50g (2oz) wholemeal breadcrumbs

Rinse the mushrooms and pat dry. Remove the stalks and chop finely, stir in the crabmeat, cheese, seasoning and chives. Preheat the grill to medium. Divide the mixture between the mushrooms, and sprinkle the top with the breadcrumbs. Place the stuffed mushrooms under grill for about 15 minutes, or until golden. Serve immediately.

SERVES 4

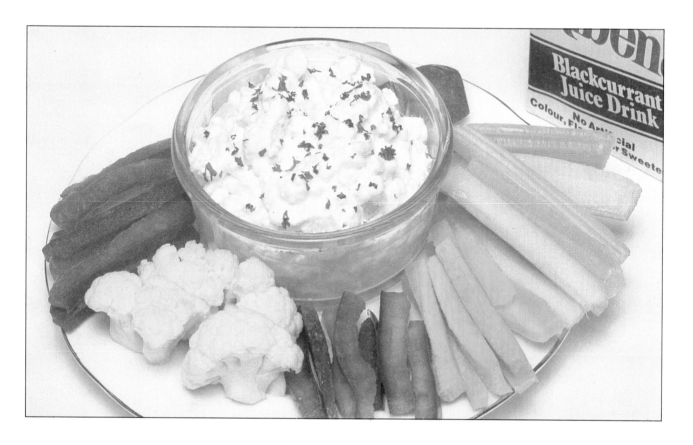

GRILLED SARDINES
220 calories per serving

2 lemons
8 fresh small sardines
50g (2oz) butter
Freshly ground pepper
2 tsp Dijon mustard
1 tsp lemon juice

Wash and cut the lemons into wedges. Wash and gut the sardines. Rinse thoroughly under running water and pat dry. Score the sardines diagonally with a knife two or three times. Preheat the grill. Meanwhile cream together the butter, pepper, mustard and lemon juice. Mash a little of this into the slits.

Grill the sardines for about 5 minutes on each side, turning carefully once. Arrange the sardines on a platter and spoon over any of the grilling sauce. Serve immediately, two sardines to a guest, with the lemon wedges and plenty of napkins!

(Pictured below)   SERVES 4

SALAD-STUFFED EGGS
115 calories per serving

4 hard-boiled eggs, shelled and halved
25g (1oz) watercress, trimmed
1 chopped spring onion
1 tbsp reduced-calorie mayonnaise
25g (1oz) cottage cheese
Cayenne
Salt and ground pepper
2 tomatoes, peeled, seeded, and very finely chopped
Large handful watercress

Remove the yolks from the eggs and set aside. Place the trimmed watercress in the bowl of a food processor with a metal blade and chop finely. Add the egg yolk, onion, mayonnaise, cottage cheese, cayenne and salt and pepper to taste. Process until smooth. Place two halves of egg white on each plate. Fill each half with a finely chopped tomato. Spoon over the egg yolk filling and mark decoratively. Place the watercress around each plate.

SERVES 4

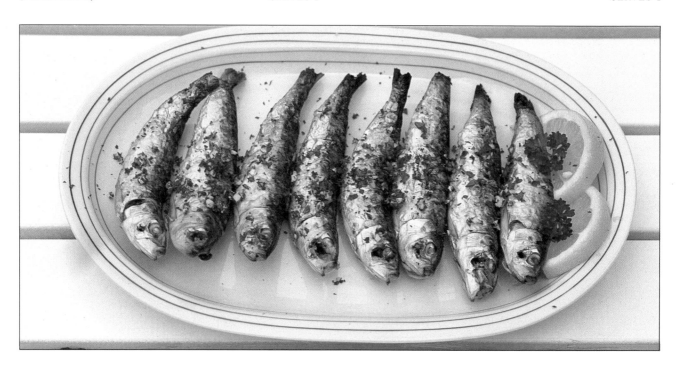

MAIN COURSES

SMOKEY SPINACH AND MACKEREL
——— *200 calories per serving* ———

450g (1lb) fresh spinach, washed and drained
Salt and pepper
350g (12oz) smoked mackerel fillets, skinned

SAUCE
250ml (½pt) skimmed milk
5 peppercorns
1 clove garlic, crushed
1 small onion, quartered
1 bay leaf
¼ nutmeg
15g (½oz) butter
100g (4oz) mushrooms, cleaned and chopped
3 spring onions, chopped
2 tbsp flour
1 tsp lemon juice
1 tsp Dijon mustard
1 tsp tomato purée

Begin by starting to make the sauce. Place the skimmed milk, peppercorns, garlic, onion, bay leaf and nutmeg in a saucepan and leave to sit for 1 hour. Meanwhile place the spinach with the water clinging to its leaves in a large saucepan, cover, and steam until wilted, stirring a little, for about 5–8 minutes. Press out the excess moisture, season, and line a baking dish with the spinach. Flake the mackerel and scatter it over the spinach.

Place the saucepan with the milk over the heat and bring to the boil. Turn down and pour the milk through a strainer into a bowl. Rinse and dry the saucepan and return to the heat. Melt the butter gently in it, then add the mushrooms and spring onions and cook until soft, about 3 minutes. Sprinkle over the flour and stir to combine and cook lightly, about 3 minutes. Gradually add the spiced milk, stirring with a whisk to avoid lumps. When all

the milk has been added, increase the heat and bring the sauce to the boil, stirring, then reduce the heat. Simmer for a few minutes until the sauce is thickened. Remove from the heat, and stir in the lemon juice, mustard and tomato purée and adjust seasoning, if necessary. Pour the sauce over the fish and spinach, and bake in a preheated 190°C/375°F/Gas 5 oven for 20–25 minutes, until bubbling. Serve with wholewheat toast points (about 60 calories per whole slice, cut into 4 points.)

SERVES 4

CHINESE SCALLOPS
——— *325 calories per serving* ———

900g (2lb) scallops, halved if large
4 tbsp flour
Ground pepper
2.5cm (1in) piece ginger, peeled and thinly sliced
2 tbsp butter
4 tbsp dry sherry

Dredge the scallops in the flour, seasoned to taste with pepper. Quickly sauté the ginger slices with the butter in a large frying pan. Add the scallops and fry them turning frequently, until they are all opaque. Add the sherry to the pan, and stir until it has been reduced to a glaze. Serve the scallops with Chinese egg noodles (200 calories per serving of 50g/2oz noodles, weighed before boiling) and a light green salad.

SERVES 4

SPICED CHICKEN WITH KUMQUATS

——— 240 calories per serving ———

2 tbsp sunflower oil
1.5kg (3½lb) chicken, skinned and cut into 8
1 clove garlic, crushed
1 tsp cinnamon
1 tsp powdered ginger
1 tsp ground coriander
Grated rind and juice of 1 orange
240ml (8fl oz) chicken stock
175g (6oz) kumquats
Salt and pepper
Fresh coriander sprigs

Preheat the oven to 180°C/350°F/Gas 4. Heat the oil in a large frying pan, add the chicken pieces and sauté over medium heat until browned lightly on both sides. Transfer the pieces to an ovenproof casserole.

Pour off most of the oil from the pan, add the garlic and cook for 1 minute. Stir in the spices, then add the orange rind, juice and stock. Allow to simmer, then add the kumquats, and seasoning to taste. Pour over the chicken and cook in the oven for about 45 minutes, or until the chicken is tender when pierced with a fork. At the last minute, stir in a few coriander leaves, and serve on a large platter, garnished with more coriander leaves. Allow two pieces per person and serve, if desired, with brown rice (90 calories per 25g/1oz uncooked – allow 50g/2oz per serving).

(Pictured below) SERVES 4

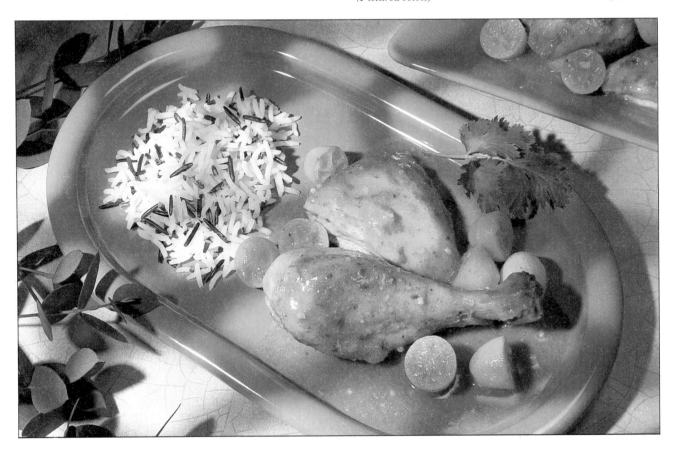

CHICKEN PSEUDO-HOLLANDAISE

— 260 calories per serving —

1 small onion, chopped
5 sprigs fresh tarragon
4 large chicken breasts
Juice of ½ lemon

SAUCE
5 large egg yolks
5 tbsp lemon juice
175ml (6fl oz) chicken broth
2 tbsp butter, melted
Salt and ground pepper
Cayenne pepper
2 tbsp Meaux or large-grain mustard

Make the sauce first. Place the egg yolks and 1 tablespoon of the lemon juice in the bowl of a food processor or blender; process with the metal blade for 1 minute. Add the remaining lemon juice to the chicken broth in a saucepan and bring to the boil. Boil until the liquid is reduced by one-third. Turn the machine back on and slowly pour in the hot liquid. When it is thoroughly combined, pour the sauce back into the saucepan and warm over very low heat until the sauce thickens, about 2 minutes. Take off the heat and whisk in the butter, salt, pepper and cayenne to taste, and the mustard. Allow to stand.

Place the onion, 1 sprig of tarragon and 240ml (8fl oz) water in a large saucepan. Add the chicken breasts, skin-side down, and the lemon juice. Bring to the boil, then reduce the heat and cover. Simmer for about 10 minutes, until the chicken is poached. Remove the chicken pieces and skin them and bone them carefully. Place a breast on each of four plates and garnish with a sprig of tarragon. Surround with the thickened Hollandaise. (Serve with boiled new potatoes, 80 calories per 100g/4oz portion.)

SERVES 4

GRILLED TROUT WITH LEMON AND BABY POTATOES

— 325 calories per serving —

4 trout, about 225g (8oz) each, cleaned and gutted
Salt and ground pepper
4 tbsp olive oil
Fresh tarragon sprigs
3 lemons
450g (1lb) new potatoes
Parsley

Rinse and dry the trout. Sprinkle it inside and out with seasoning to taste. Cut two diagonal slashes on each side to allow heat to penetrate. Moisten each trout with 1 tsp oil, then stuff the inside of each with a few tarragon sprigs. Squeeze the juice of half a lemon over each trout, using two lemons in all. Preheat the grill to medium and grill the trout for about 5 minutes a side, turning gently once.

Meanwhile, cook the new potatoes in boiling water until tender: drain thoroughly. Serve one trout and 100g (4oz) new potatoes to each person, garnished with parsley and a quarter lemon.

SERVES 4

FRUITY SEAFISH ROLLS
300 calories per serving

2 pink grapefruit
2 shallots, finely chopped
150ml (¼pt) dry white wine
4 medium trout or 2 small bass, filleted and skinned
2 tbsp chopped fresh dill
Salt and pepper
40g (1½oz) butter
1 clove garlic, chopped
350g (12oz) courgettes, cut into matchsticks
1 tsp cornflour
Dill to garnish

Grate the rind from one of the grapefruit and put it into a baking dish, together with the shallots and wine. Cut away the peel and pith from both the grapefruits, and then cut out the segments, holding the fruit over the baking dish to catch the juice. Place the segments in a bowl.

Place the fish fillets in the baking dish with the marinade; if you are using the bass, cut each fillet in two. Marinate the fish for half an hour. Reserve 8 of the grapefruit segments and chop the remainder.

Preheat the oven to 190°C/375°F/Gas 5. Remove the fillets from the marinade, place on a board skin-side down, and scatter over the chopped dill. Season to taste and divide the chopped grapefruit among the fillets. Roll up each piece of fish and put into an ovenproof dish, pour over the marinade and dot with the butter. Cover and bake for 15 minutes.

Meanwhile heat the remaining butter in a frying pan, add the garlic and cook for 1 minute. Add the courgettes and heat lightly until only just cooked. Arrange the courgettes on a serving platter with the trout and reserved grapefruit segments. Return the dish to the oven to keep warm. Strain the cooking juices into a saucepan and simmer for 2 minutes. Blend the cornflour with a tablespoon of water, add to the pan and cook the sauce until thickened. Pour a little sauce over the fish rolls, garnish with the dill and serve the rest separately.

(Pictured right) SERVES 4

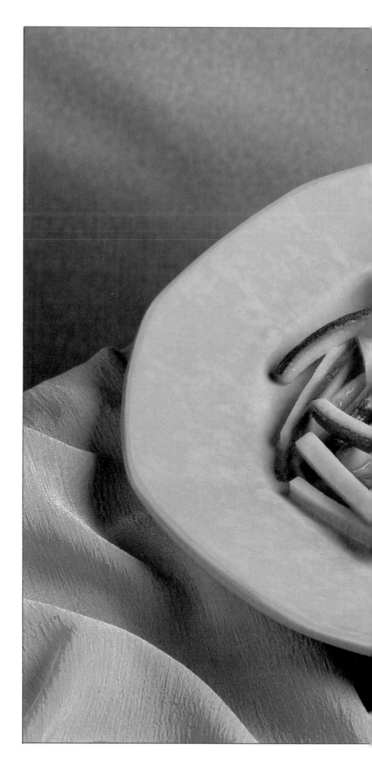

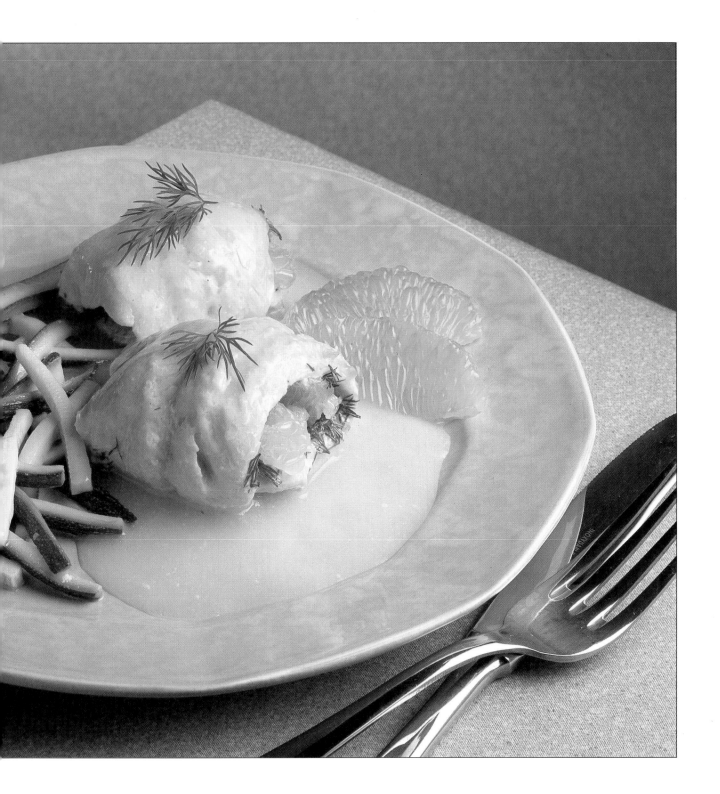

OCCASIONAL DESSERTS

Although we know that it is easy enough to gain weight or eat unhealthily without indulging in desserts and sweet things, it is usually this 'extra' which is among the first to go when you are trying to keep to a low-calorie, low-fat regime. This is because desserts almost always contain sugar and/or dairy fat, both of which are calorie-killers. However, sometimes a dessert is called for – as at a dinner party – or just wanted – because you've been good for so long! The recipes below are all surprisingly low in the sugar and fat stakes, largely because they are based on fresh fruit – hardly naughty and very nice!

EXOTIC TERRINE WITH VANILLA SAUCE
210 calories per serving

Juice of 2 oranges
40g (1½oz) powdered gelatin
3 tbsp caster sugar
900ml (1½pt) sparkling white grape juice
250g (12oz) strawberries
1 kiwi fruit, peeled and sliced
1 ripe, firm mango, peeled and sliced

SAUCE
1 vanilla pod
1 tsp cornflour
280ml (½pt) milk
2 egg yolks
25g (1oz) caster sugar
3 tbsp single cream

Place the orange juice into a bowl, sprinkle over the gelatin and allow it to soak in. Place the bowl in a pan of simmering water, and stir until the gelatin has dissolved. Add the sugar and stir until it too has dissolved. Set aside to cool slightly.

Slowly add the grape juice to the bowl and whisk. Strain the liquid into a bowl and place in a refrigerator until it begins to thicken. Skim off any surface froth.

Meanwhile choose the 8 smallest strawberries and halve them. Chop the remainder. Rinse a loaf tin with cold water and stand it in a dish surrounded by ice cubes. Pour in a little of the grape jelly over the bottom – it will thicken quickly. Arrange the sliced kiwi down the centre and the halved strawberries alongside. Spoon over a little more jelly, then cover with a layer of chopped strawberries. Continue the layers of jelly and berries until the tin is full, ending with a layer of jelly. Refrigerate to chill and set.

Make the vanilla sauce: place the vanilla pod in a saucepan and pour over the milk. Heat gently to just simmering. Turn off the heat and allow to set for a few minutes. Remove the pod. Put the cornflour into a bowl, blend with a little of the milk, beat in the egg yolks, then the sugar and the rest of the milk. Return the sauce to the saucepan and then to a low heat, stirring constantly until it is thick enough to coat a spoon. Strain the sauce into a bowl and set aside to cool. Whisk in the cream and chill.

To unmould the terrine, dip the tin into a bowl of hot water for 10 seconds, remove, and press the edges of the jelly away from the tin. Place a serving plate over the top of the terrine, invert it and give the top a tap. Serve each slice in a pool of vanilla sauce.

(Pictured opposite)   SERVES 8

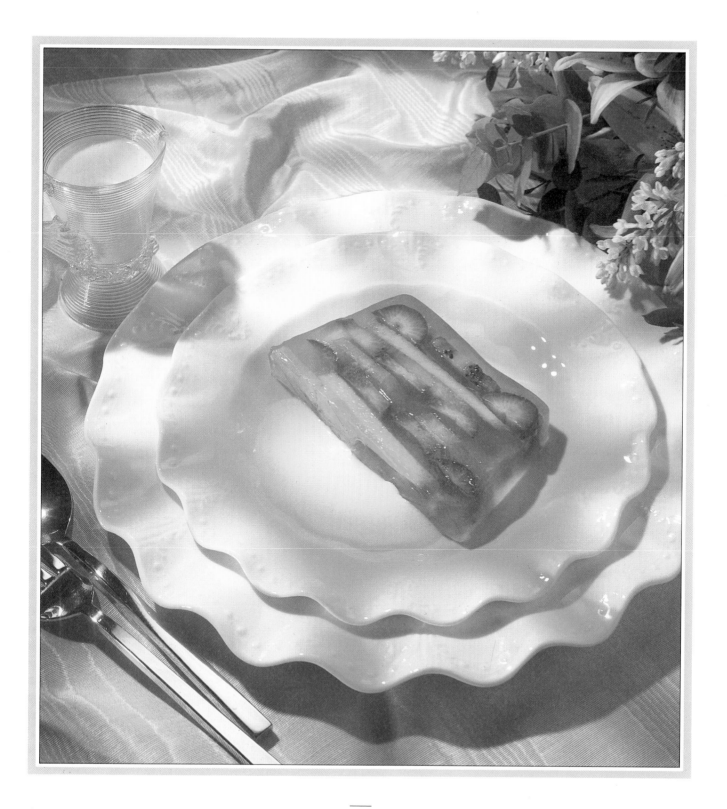

PEARS IN RED WINE
130 calories per serving

4 Anjou or Comise pears
1 tbsp fresh lemon juice
225ml (8fl oz) dry red wine
50g (2oz) caster sugar
1 stick cinnamon
5 cloves
4 allspice berries

Peel the pears, leaving the stems attached. Coat with the lemon juice.

Mix the wine, sugar, and spices in a saucepan large enough to hold the pears upright. Before adding the pears, bring the liquid to the boil. Put in the pears; if the liquid does not cover them, add a little water. Cover and simmer for about 25 minutes, or until tender. Remove the pears from the heat and allow to cool in the syrup. Remove the pears to a bowl, place the saucepan on the heat and reduce the sauce by half. Pour over the pears and chill for 4 hours or more. Serve the pears surrounded by small pools of the sauce.

SERVES 4

CARIBBEAN MANGO
110 calories per serving

3 large mangoes
Juice of 3 limes
3 tbsp honey
2 cloves

Pare the mangoes and cut the flesh away from the pit lengthwise into long slices. Divide the slices between six plates. Mix the lime juice, honey and cloves in a small bowl; drizzle over the mango pieces. Serve immediately.

SERVES 6

TURKISH FIGS
110 calories per serving

8 fresh purple figs
140ml (¼pt) 1% fromage frais
140ml (¼pt) low-fat yoghurt
4 tsp of brown sugar

Put the figs in a bowl of boiling water for 1 minute. Drain, then peel them. Slice the figs through from the stem end almost to the bottom, and again, resulting in each fruit opened like a flower into four 'petals'. Place the two figs on each plate.

Mix together the fromage frais and yoghurt. Pour some over each serving, and sprinkle a teaspoon of brown sugar over each. Chill for 2–3 hours before serving; the sugar will 'caramelise' over the yoghurt.

SERVES 4

RASPBERRY ZABAGLIONE
130 calories per serving

450g (1lb) raspberries, washed and picked over
2 egg yolks, beaten
2 tbsp sugar
3 tbsp framboise or Marsala
2 tbsp dry white wine

Save four prime raspberries, then divide the remainder between four tall glasses. Place the egg yolks in a small bowl, and half submerge it in a large saucepan of hot water. Whisk until the yolks are pale and frothy. Then whisk in the sugar, framboise or Marsala and wine. Continue to beat until the mixture is fluffy. Then spoon over the fruit in the glasses, decorate the top of each with a reserved raspberry, and serve immediately.

SERVES 4

PINK AND WHITE FRUIT KEBABS

150 calories per serving

350g (12oz) strawberries
350g (12oz) lychees, peeled and stones removed
Grated rind and juice of 1 small orange
3 tbsp white wine

SAUCE
100g (4oz) strawberries
90ml (3fl oz) strawberry fromage frais
2 tbsp double cream

Put the strawberries and lychees into a bowl, add the orange rind, juice and wine and toss together. Cover and chill for one hour. Thread the fruit onto 8 small skewers.

To make the sauce, purée the strawberries in a blender or food processor, then press through a sieve into a bowl. Add the fromage frais and 1 tsp of the fruit marinade. Whisk together until smooth.

To serve with nouvelle cuisine panache, pour a pool of strawberry sauce onto each of four plates. Add a dot of cream to each, then swirl with a knife to create a pattern. Place two kebabs attractively against the sauce.

(Pictured below)   SERVES 4

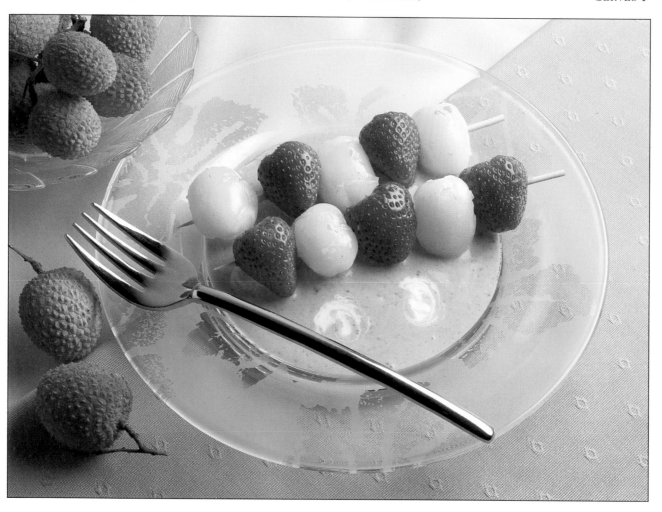

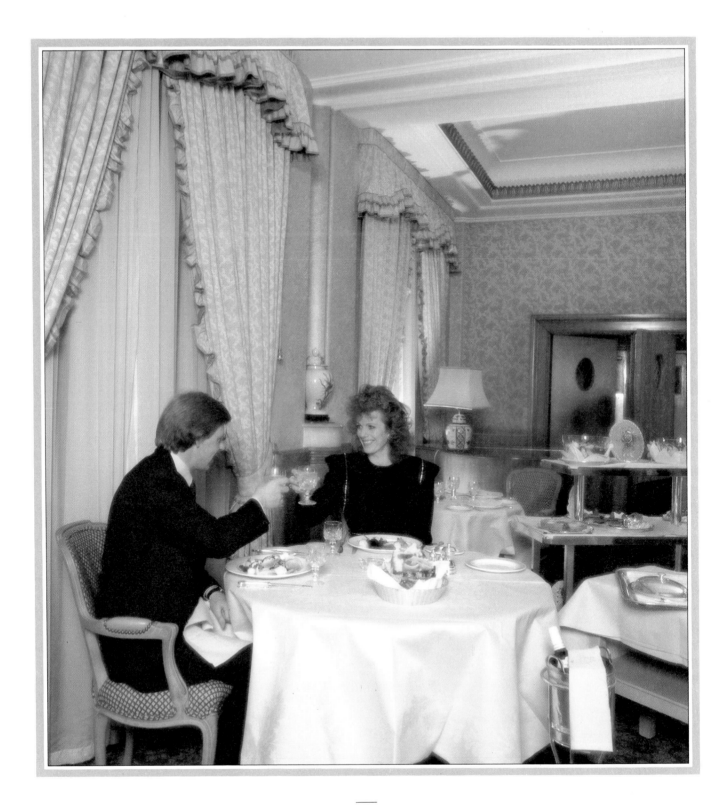

EATING OUT
and EATING WELL

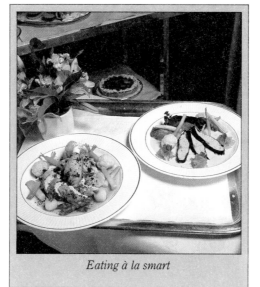

Eating à la smart

others who are usually stuck at home look forward to going out. Working men and women, whose lives revolve around the business lunch, and often an evening meal out as well, sigh for good 'home-cooked' food. We're never satisfied! But everyone seems to agree that a diet of restaurant grub can't be all that good for you somehow. Sorry frustrated homemakers – and take heart, luncheon tycoons – that's not quite true. As at home, your diet is as healthy and balanced as you make it – it's up to you.

You aren't simply at the mercy of restaurauteurs. *You* order your meals, after all. You may not be putting together the salad on your plate or cooking your main course in the kitchen, but you do have a certain control over what goes onto your plate. You know, for instance, that ordering deep-fried breaded mozzarella bites in an Italian restaurant will mean plenty of cholesterol, saturated fat and calories, and that a hefty cheeseburger on a sesame bun is rich in animal fat, protein and refined carbohydrates. Both dishes may taste scrumptious and once in a while

won't do you any harm, but foods like that eaten regularly are no basis for a healthy diet. Having a meal out, especially if you eat out a lot, needs just as much care and good sense as planning a meal in. You just have the hard work done for you.

If you generally only go out as a treat, a commitment to healthy eating will mean that you want to choose dishes that build on the good work you have carried on at home. And if you do eat out regularly, you definitely should take an active interest in eating better restaurant food. Follow a mental checklist of the points we covered on pages 10 to 14 and apply the criteria to dishes that appeal on the menu.

1 Look for dishes that are low in saturated fats – indeed as low in all fats as possible. This means concentrating on fish, poultry and vegetarian dishes and cutting down on red meat; avoiding creamy, cheesy or buttery sauces and fried foods; and eliminating salads with fattening ingredients such as bacon, nuts, cheese and egg.
2 If you are avoiding fried food, it follows that you should be seeking out the best methods of

cooking noted on the menu. Look out for grilled and steamed foods – fish and vegetables taste especially fresh and true prepared this way.

3 Try to steer away from foods which are based on sugar, and avoid dishes which are likely to be salty, such as crisps, chips, sausages etc. This is a particular risk at fast food outlets and cafés, and with pub lunches, in which many of the prepared hot dishes can be oversalted. As for sugary desserts, avoid syrupy puddings, mousses, gateaux and most pastries. Move towards fresh fruit salads, berries or fruits with a topping of yogurt (rather than cream), or even the occasional banana flambé or strawberries in champagne.

4 Avoiding fatty and sugary foods releases calories which can be more usefully directed toward the complex carbohydrates. Rid yourself of the outmoded fear that pasta, potatoes and rice *per se* are bad for you: remember it's the butter, bolognese and piles of cheese you put on them that does the damage. If you stick to vegetable sauces, or the slightly richer seafood sauces (*sans* cheese and cream), you should be OK.

Of course, wholemeal versions of pasta and rice are even better – they have exactly the same calorific value as their refined relatives, but greater nutritive value. *And* they fill you up more – which is useful when the dessert trolley comes round. But facing facts as they are now, it is unlikely that you will encounter many offers of wholemeal pasta and rice on the restaurant circuit; they are considered too chewy for the 'average' palate and take too long to cook. But cafés and restaurant which style themselves 'wholefood' have a selection of hot and cold dishes based on them, usually combined with equally healthy vegetarian sauces and dressings.

5 As mentioned in (1), vegetables should play a larger part in a healthy diet, even when out on the town or at a business lunch. Look for first courses like vegetable-based soups (without cream), whole fresh artichokes or asparagus, or leeks, mushrooms or other vegetables served à la greque. Whenever possible, choose dishes based on raw vegetables, such as crudités, tomatoes with vinaigrette dressing or a composed salad. Try not to adulterate such healthy basics with too rich a dressing. If possible, ask for it to be omitted or served separately so that you can help yourself – to a minimum!

6 Don't fall into the bread-nibbler's trap. This is hard, since on a busy day you will sometimes have to wait quite a while for the waiter to take your order or for the arrival of the food. Meanwhile, there it is – that tempting little basket of bread, often very *tasty* bread, that comes with the cover charge, just sitting there waiting to be picked at. And then there is that tub of lovely unsalted butter that spreads so well and tastes sooo yummy. Two temptations! Resist them!! Remember that every piece of chunky restaurant-style bread is likely to have 80–110 calories, while butter is a staggering 210 calories an ounce. Save yourself for the serious business of eating.

7 Treat alcohol with care. The average glass of wine contains between 90–100 calories, and it is difficult to stop at one when you are having a good meal. A few glasses of wine also seem to justify a splurge on the main dishes, and may make it harder to say no when the orders for dessert come round. It's all part of the 'letting go' syndrome.

Of course, if it is a celebration or a special night out, 'a little of what you fancy does you good', but try to keep the consumption down. For business lunches, it should be easier, since drinking in the middle of a working day isn't the best idea in any case. Most restaurants, even local 'pit stops', sell still and sparkling mineral waters, and fruit juices are another healthy option.

8 Finally, to conclude on a healthy note, try to avoid coffee at the end of the meal. Coffee has been blamed for increasing the pulse rate and for interfering with the efficiency of the digestive process. One alternative is to order decaffeinated coffee, which certainly is an improvement on the original version. Another, even better, choice is a herb tea such as peppermint, camomile, fennel or verbena. They have a tonic effect, helping digestion and calming the nerves. Some people swear by a mixture of hot water and lemon taken as a *digestif*. A popular drink among healthy Italian restaurant-goers, it is sometimes called a 'canary'.

After these general guidelines, it may be helpful to go on to review some of the most popular cuisines and eating places. Every type of restaurant and café will have something to appeal to the health-conscious customer – though, in some places, like pubs and snack bars, you may have to look a little harder. But with increasing public awareness of what good eating means, it is becoming easier and easier to eat out without compromising your health.

TRADITIONAL BRITISH FARE

Nowadays 'Traditional English' can mean anything from the roasts and bread-and-butter puddings of old establishments like Rules or Simpson's to the *nouvelle Britannique* cuisine of some of the newer, trendier restaurants. In the latter, there are often vegetarian or 'healthy eating' dishes starred in the menu. Lacking this, among the healthier, lower-calorie choices to be found on an English-style *carte* are:

Consommés of beef, chicken, pheasant or game, and thin soups such as cock-a-leekie. Fresh vegetable soups also feature on some menus – but delicious as they are you should try to limit those made with cream (such as lettuce and asparagus).

First courses such as asparagus (choose vinaigrette rather than butter, or better yet, fresh lemon to be squeezed over); oysters (almost *no* calories, but watch out for the buttered brown bread!); soused and smoked fish (the soused fish – usually herring – is lower in calories than the smoked, but both are fairly light); fish and vegetable terrines (though usually made with cream, you get very little in a slice); quails' eggs (*without* mayonnaise); and stuffed or marinated vegetables.

Main courses include fish, poultry and game dishes – particularly those which are steamed or grilled. Salmon and sole are, of course, favourite stars of the national table and are both delicious when prepared in this way. Duck is best avoided, but chicken, pheasant, partridge, guinea fowl and even venison are low-caloried alternatives, provided they are not richly sauced.

The British are not renowned for their light desserts – they're not generically called 'puddings' for nothing. If you succumb, go for fresh strawberries, fruit salad or, at the outside, a fruit crumble (all without cream, of course!)

FRENCH AND INTERNATIONAL

Many of the same dishes are offered on the French menu as on the up-market English menu, except, of course, they've got French names. Items like smoked salmon (usually from Scotland or Ireland when served in the UK and the Loire when served in France), oyster, artichokes and asparagus, are regular first course features on French and international menus – and whether in English or a foreign language they are good choices for the figure- and health-conscious. Other options include soups like consommés, and wonderful vegetable soups – though make sure that cream is not included. Terrines and pâtés are both creations of *haute cuisine* – keep

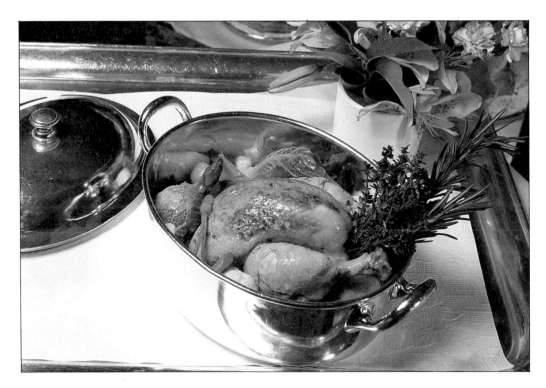

*An excellent choice –
plump chicken poached
with fresh vegetables*

away from those which are based on offal and pork – good substitutes are light chicken terrines, fish and vegetable versions. Again, all will contain some cream, but a thin slice should do little harm. The same is not true for mousses, however, which usually have a higher proportion of cream. Ask for brown-bread toast and leave off the butter!

Crudités are a French invention that have caught on all over – crunchy carrots, spring onions, cauliflower, mushrooms, celery, red and green peppers and other raw vegetables, accompanied by a tangy dipping sauce. Unless the sauce is yoghurt-based, treat it warily. Most are mayonnaise-based and quite high in calories. It's actually best if you can keep away from the dip altogether, and concentrate on the fresh bite of the unadulterated vegetables! *Moules* (mussels) are a more adventurous course – while they are high in cholesterol, they are very

low in calories, as long as they are not bathed in a rich sauce. Stick to *moules marinière* (which should be made without any cream, though many restaurants cheat. Ask first). A favourite of 'international' restaurants is prawn cocktail. Though prawns are low in calories, they are then smothered in a dressing loaded with them. Ask for the prawns *without* the dressing and for extra lemon wedges. You'll be surprised at how honest they taste!

If you are electing to have fish as your main course, bravo! Fish in general is much lower in calories, and in animal fat. Grilled or steamed fish are your best bet; try to avoid the saucy dishes with the elegant names – Waleska, Veronique, Bonne Femme, etc – all smothered in butter and cream. Let the fish speak for itself. As for types of fish, some are actually lower in calories and fat then others – the best are oysters, crab, lobster, mussels, cod, halibut, haddock, plaice, prawns and shrimp, sole, trout, fresh tuna and turbot; the *very* lowest in calories are cod, mussels, oysters, plaice, sole and trout. If you are on a strict diet, leave the salmon, mackerel, kippers and herring for the moment.

It is when you come to meats and poultry in the French or 'international' style that the calories and animal fat begin to mount. As the old chestnut goes, the French are fond of sauces – usually based on wine, cream and butter, flavoured with fruit, herbs or cheese. Avoid these and go for the grilled items – possibles are poussins or chicken breast, game such as pheasant, partridge or guinea fowl, or, if you don't have ethical qualms, lean veal. The ubiquitous breast of duck is often a good choice when presented French-style, since the piece is usually thinly-sliced, so not very large, and well-trimmed of fat. Scrape off the excess sauce.

If the meal you are attacking is lunch, or if you prefer a lighter dinner, it is becoming more and more acceptable (indeed fashionable!) to eat two first courses and do away with the traditional entrée. This means that you can follow a delicate vegetable terrine with a composed salad, or artichoke vinaigrette with a bowl of mussels. French restaurants particularly lend themselves to this kind of combination, and the staff seem quite happy to oblige. After all, that's how all those elegant French women keep their figures! This is also a good ploy for vegetarians. Although the French are not big on vegetarian cuisine as such, their hors d'oeuvres usually cover a large gamut of toothsome vegetable-based dishes.

If you must have something to end the meal, be very French and elect cheese *without* biscuits. Best choices are lower-fat cheeses such as Bel Paese, Edam, Gouda, Brie and Camembert. If you fancy a blue cheese, chose Roquefort over Stilton – the difference is 40 calories an ounce! Otherwise stick to fresh fruit – strawberries, pineapple slices, figs – fruit salad or fruit crêpes (ask them to lay off the sugar!). All of these, needless to say, without cream. Forego the sweet wines and liqueurs as well – the healthy French often do!

ITALIAN RESTAURANTS AND PIZZA PARLOURS

Italian food has a reputation for being a dieter's foe – but that is largely the fault of all-you-can-eat pasta pig-out places which pile on the Bolognese sauce. Authentic Italian cooking can be very healthy – witness the relatively low incidence of heart disease in the Italian peninsula – and makes great use of fresh vegetables. The secret is not to get carried away with the yumminess of it all and order too much.

In addition to consommé, Italian low-calorie soup options include straciatella (really consommé with thin-egg stands in it) and minestrone. Both are lower in calories than practically any other first course you might pick – if they are enjoyed without buttered rolls. As for more substantial choices, health-conscious Italian appetizers include parma ham with or without melon, fresh grapefruit, *insalata de mare* (seafood salad largely composed of low-caloried squid), and mozzarella and tomato salad. Keep away from the deep-fried dishes: mozzarella in bread, whitebait, mushrooms and stuffed courgette flowers, all of which rate high in the fat stakes because of the batter and the deep-frying method, as well as because of the stuffings and dips which are part of many of the recipes.

Much-maligned pasta can actually be very good for you if the sauce is not rich. But the problem in restaurants, in addition to ordering the right sauce, is making sure you don't eat too much. Helpings in most places are pretty large, and if you are having first *and* second courses, it is very easy to overdo the calorie count. If you really do love your pasta, it is probably best to allow yourself to indulge in a sensible pasta for your main course. 'Sensible pastas' include spaghetti, fettucine or linguine served with a sauce napoletana (with tomato, onion, basil and garlic), marinara (with seafood, tomato and garlic), vongole (with white wine, tomatoes and clams), or al tonno (with wine and tuna). Vegetable lasagna or cannelloni are sometimes offered and would do especially well as a main course choice. Parmesan is a rich cheese at 130 calories an ounce, so try to hold back on nodding too enthusiastically when the waiter comes round with his spoon and bowl of cheese. It may help to remember that it is classically correct *not* to serve Parmesan with fish-based pastas like marinara, tonno and vongole, though many gutsy people can't resist it!

Pizza is not one of the lowest-calorie dishes you might order, but ounce-for-ounce it can be quite healthy if made with the right ingredients. It should be a real yeast dough, the base thick compared to the filling (in other words, stay away from deep-dish!), and covered with fresh tomato sauce. Eliminate toppings which are primarily cheese or meat – go for fresh tomatoes, vegetables, onions, tuna and anchovies. If wholemeal crust is available, try it. It's no lower in calories, but it's higher in fibre and unrefined carbohydrates.

Italian main courses tend toward the heavy, but careful choosing repays. Fish are not usually offered in styles suitable to the health-conscious. Keep away from the deep-fried scampi and mixed seafood and the numberless fish in wine and butter sauces. Go for the grilled sole or trout. As for meat and poultry, concentrate on the roast and grilled birds, especially quail, pheasant and chicken diavolo (usually poussin devilled and grilled). Avoid those dishes wrapped in cheese and tomato sauce.

Italian dessert cheeses tend to be creamier than their French counterpart, and therefore higher in calories. Better to opt for fresh fruit or Italian sorbet – most other Italian desserts are notoriously naughty.

AMERICAN-STYLE EATERIES

Hamburger joints and up-market American-style restaurants have been spreading all over Britain in the last few years, and their food has been getting more authentic and better all the time – at least in terms of taste. In terms of healthy eating, the staples of American diners and fast-food outlets have never been known for their goodness. Hamburgers, oozing with fatty juices, bathed in mayonnaise and ketchup and partnered by a mountain of French fries, are hardly the stuff superman – or woman – is made of. The options here for the seriously concerned eater are pretty limited.

First courses are probably down to vegetable soup or corn-on-the-cob without salt or butter. Close your eyes to that garlic bread literally squelching in butter!

If you must have a hamburger, have it grilled and off the bun. If red meat is really what you want, you would be even better off with a well-trimmed steak. But there are a few other, better choices if you have the will-power to make them. One obvious alternative to the hamburger is a sandwich – try chopped chicken or tuna on wholewheat; ask them to go easy on the mayo. Most 'American' restaurants offer barbecued chicken – this will be about the lowest-calorie possibility you will see among the hot choices. If given the choice as to potato, order baked rather than chips; don't smother it in butter but use small amounts of the proffered sour cream.

The other safe options will be cold: chef's salad or perhaps a salad niçoise. Though the latter is hardly American, it has been adopted with alacrity by many of these places. With any salad, ask for the dressing to be served separately and use sparingly. (And stay away from the luscious Caesar salad – the calories lurking in the Parmesan, egg yolk, oil and garlic croutons are alarming.)

Finally, dessert. American desserts must be among the most sinful in the world, their development a reaction against that pilgrim puritan ethic. Milk shakes, fudge sundaes, brownies, banana splits, mocha mud pie, devil's food cake – the names are enough to provoke a cardiac arrest. You may find yourself falling when you enter this den of iniquity, and one once in a while won't kill you. But if you want to stay pure, desist entirely or at the most succumb to apple pie, unenhanced by cream or ice cream.

SPANISH AND MEXICAN CASAS

These are the new boys on the stylish restaurant scene – a few years ago they were few and far between. Among the Spanish restaurants, the most popular and stylish are the *tapas* bars, in which a selection of large 'snacks' are offered across the bar, and customers usually order several among a group to sample with wine or sherry. Mexican restaurants, on the other hand, specialize in the country fare of southwestern and northern Mexico – spicy dishes composed largely of pork, beef or chicken, rolled up in corn or flour tortillas.

Of the two, the tapas bar offers the greater choice to the weight- and health-conscious; dishes usually include low-calorie grilled or marinated shrimp, mushrooms, squid, sardine bites, chicken wings, and tomato toasts. Keep away from olives (at 5 calories an olive, they mount up quickly), the meatballs, quiches or omelettes, and items with grilled cheese. Since drink is the focus of the exercise, you may want a glass or two (preferably of dry white wine), but the sooner you can move onto mineral water

the better. Evenings like this have a way of going on!

The Mexican restaurant options, like those of Northern American, are fairly limited. A likely soup might be gazpacho (actually Spanish in origin, but found in many Latin restaurants), a first course ripe avocado served simply with fresh lime. Seviche (a dish of raw fish marinated in lime juice which 'cooks' it) is a possibility low in calories but very high in 'good things'.

In the main courses, steer away from the various stuffed tortillas, some deep-fried and others not, but all topped with loads of sour cream, guacamole and cheese. If you must have one, the best choice would probably be the bean buritto – and ask them to hold the extras. Otherwise you would do well to keep your eyes fixed on the grilled fish and chicken, boring as they may seem in comparison.

When it comes to desserts, it is not as difficult to say no the those of Spain and Mexico as it is to those of some other countries. Fruit is fine!

INDIAN RESTAURANTS

Indian restaurants are among the most beloved and patronised of all Britain's many ethnic establishments. So it behooves the healthy eater to assess the Indian menu for the best options, since chances are circumstances, friends and hunger will take him or her there sooner rather than later!

Generally speaking, the tandoori specialities will be lower in calories and fat than the saucy curries, with their sometime additives of cream, egg, ground almonds and coconut. Of the first courses, therefore, the chicken tikka and kebabs are the health leaders, while prawn patia is a slightly moister alternative. If you are not having a first course, a couple of plain pompaddums are an acceptable indulgence, but don't get carried away – and don't allow yourself to start dipping in the chutneys!

On to the main courses, which again lean to chicken and prawn tandooris. Mutton is fattier and more calorific. Some sophisticated restaurants offer other tandoori-cooked food, such as fish (usually bass) and quail. Both of these are very good choices. If you do want curry, it is lowest in calories to stick to the vegetable varieties. But if you crave something more substantial, choose prawn or at a pinch, chicken – and preferably one of the drier versions, such as Bhuna or Madras or, even better, a Biriyani. Dhansak, Masala, Kashmiri and Korma are all too rich for someone who is seriously trying to keep the weight down. Try to split the rice, nan or chapati with someone – and keep away from the fried parathas! Indian yoghurt is not as low-calorie as you might expect either. It is made from whole fat milk and is thick and creamy. So don't treat it as if it's a harmless filler.

Like Mexican cuisine, it should not be difficult to say no to the rather sweet and sickly Indian desserts. And drink mineral water rather than the inevitable lager.

TURKISH AND GREEK TAVERNAS

These restaurants do really not cater for vegetarians, and the choice of items based on this reliably low-calorie foodstuff is somewhat limited. Low calorie first-course options include tzaziki (yoghurt and cucumber) with a *little* pitta (125 calories a pitta!) or a Greek salad. Taramasalata and hummus are both oily and rich. Entrée choices like grilled red mullet or prawns, when available, should be taken advantage of. Otherwise it's the inevitable kebab – chicken, if possible. Stews and moussakas are usually quite high in calories.

Bakalava and the other phyllo, nut and honey desserts are very high in calories – around 250 per small piece – so succumb at your peril!

ORIENTAL RESTAURANTS

Oriental restaurants offer some of the widest variety of healthy, low-fat, low-caloried food to the adventurous eater. They begin with a headstart, since they do not use butter, cream or cheese in their cooking – in fact, cheese is regarded as rotten milk!

Probably the leading cuisine on the flab-fighting front is the Japanese. The soups are delicious broths, while the Japanese make great use of fish, both cooked and raw. Traditional Japanese cooking does not have three or four courses as we do, but rather has five distinctive types of dishes – raw, grilled, simmered, stewed or fried – which are presented in a customary order. However, modern restaurant etiquette enables diners to order the types of dishes they like in any number or combination. Seaweed and pickled vegetables also appear. Almost any Japanese dish – except for the deep-fried tempura – is a good one for the discerning eater. Sushi – raw fish wrapped round or over vinegared rice, with or without seaweed – is probably the healthiest, lowest-caloried dish you will find in any restaurant, ethnic or otherwise.

Chinese food runs the gamut – from the healthy fish and vegetable soups, steamed fish and rice, and quick-cooked shellfish and stir-frys, all of which are good choices for the figure-conscious – to the calorie-laden sticky spare ribs, deep-fried batter prawns and spring rolls, and glutinous sweet-and-sour sauced dishes. This, of course, is the Cantonese cuisine, the one most frequently encountered. Other variations – Pekinese and Schezwan among them – offer other options like a greater variety of baked and highly-spiced dishes.

Try to keep the fried foods to a minimum, though unlike Western-style frying, it's done at such a high temperature and so quickly that little fat actually penetrates the food. Concentrate on

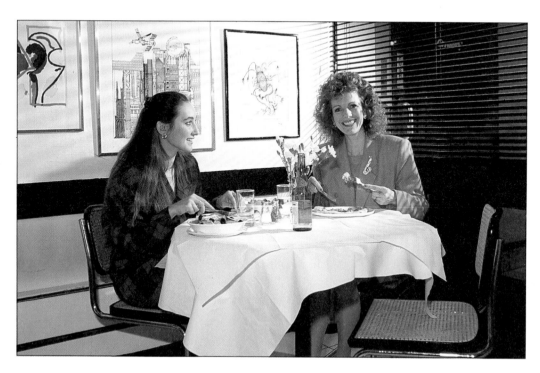

You can eat well and stay slim!

the wealth of fish dishes available – from steamed ginger crab in the shell to wonderful whole baked fish dishes. Vary the order with a few vegetable dishes and steamed rice.

Finally, there are all the burgeoning East Asian cuisines on the scene: Thai, Vietnamese, Malaysian and Singaporean. All of these nationalities glorify the realms of fish and vegetables, and all use relatively healthful methods of cooking them – steaming, grilling, and quick stir-frying. Chicken and pork also feature – both usually prepared as healthily as possible, though you would be best advised to stick to chicken for calorie reasons. Keep away from the varieties of 'hot-pot' cooking, unless it is fish to be table-cooked in a court bouillon. The beef and pork versions are less lightweight. Keep away from the fried batter and won-ton pastry dishes and ask for steamed or boiled rice.

For an exotic change, and one comparatively low in calories, try a spicy shellfish soup or one of the seafood noodle dishes. These have a full complement of hot peppers, lime and lemon grass, as well as rich coconut milk or coconut itself. But the complexity of flavours and heat of the spice means that they are quite filling in relation to the amount you eat. You will find yourself well satisfied by one dish rather than succumbing to the temptation of eating several smaller dishes that eventually mount up!

Another favourite, particularly of Malaysian and Thai restaurants, are the cooked 'salads'. These are an alternative healthy choice, particularly if they are seafood or chicken-based.

PUB FOOD AND SNACK BARS

There are occasions when a fully-fledged lunch out is just not on. Business has to be discussed over a drink in the pub, with food quickly snatched at the bar, or an even more hurried lunch grabbed at your desk between meetings.

This is when knowing what is value-for-calories can really pay off.

Sandwiches are often the easiest and most varied choice available at the local snack bar. Gone are the days when a British sandwich meant two dried and curled slices of white bread with an indeterminate piece of pinkish meat lost somewhere in between. The place of the sandwich in a healthy lifestyle has been vindicated – as long as you follow a few simple guidelines. Go for wholewheat and grain breads every time; make sure that they are not lacquered with butter and laden with high-fat fillings. Most sandwich bars will use low-fat spreads if you request it – and it is possible to ask for fillings in which little, if any, spread is needed at all. Try instead moist fillings like prawn and cottage cheese, mashed tuna (which will probably have some salad cream in it already) or mashed sardine with lettuce, or tomato and scrambled egg. Or order thin-sliced boiled ham with mustard, or a sandwich of cooked, skinned chicken, of plain tuna, or of sliced tomato, cucumber and lettuce, and buy a small pot of plain low-fat yoghurt – you can use that as a spread when you are back at your desk. Steer clear of cream cheese and hard cheeses; beef, pastrami and most other meats; coleslaw, egg salad and other mayonnaise-bound fillings. Avoid quiches, pasties and meat pies, but don't be shy of the ubiquitous baked potato.

In both pubs and take-aways, the baked potato has become a fixture. This has not done much to improve its reputation as a heavy, high-calorie food, which is certainly undeserved. Like pasta, it is what you put on it that makes the difference. Loads of butter and grated cheese are *not* the optimum choice, nor is chilli con carne, mountains of sour cream or curry. Instead ask for cottage cheese and prawns, tuna and sweetcorn, or yoghurt with chopped chives. An average baked potato will set you back a mere 180–200 calories and, with a sensible filling added, about 300. That's not bad for a nutritious, warming and satisfying meal.

The choice of other healthy hot meals in a pub may be fairly limited. The flour-thickened curries, greasy hot pots and lasagnes, sausages and mash, or ersatz shepherd's pie won't do much for your waistline or fatty lipid count. If the pub offers a vegetarian option like cauliflower cheese, ratatouille or a vegetable curry, take it. Chicken or scampi in a basket, with a garnish of tomato and lettuce, are acceptable runners-up. Low-calorie sandwiches are always OK.

LAST ORDERS

This about ends our ramble through the wide world of restaurants, cafés, bistros, brasseries, snack bars and pubs. I have probably missed a few esoteric cuisines and no doubt some of the possibilities you'll see chalked up on the blackboard or down in the menus, but you've got the general idea by now. Once you get in the habit of really noticing what you eat, and expecting from the restaurants the same care for quality and 'real food' value you try to achieve at home, making the healthy choice becomes second nature. This is not to say that eating out must become a test, or analyzing the menu a bore. On the contrary, your heightened awareness should help you to appreciate your food more while fueling your system with the best 'high-octane petrol' the market offers. And for 'lead-free' read 'low-fat' – something every sensitive and alert driver in the fast lane of life knows is important!

A last realistic piece of advice. Remember that if you have strayed from the sensible paths of nutrition on occasion – panic not!

The *occasional* over-indulgence on the odd night out – when 'a *lot* of what you fancy' has taken precedence over your normal eating habits – matters not. Just make sure you balance it the next day by enjoying a bigger portion of vegetables and fruit. Your body fuel makes your engine tick over, and it's good to know that the majority of the time it is being well and truly fed in the best possible way!

Cheers and Happy Eating!

TOTAL HEALTH & FITNESS

EXERCISE

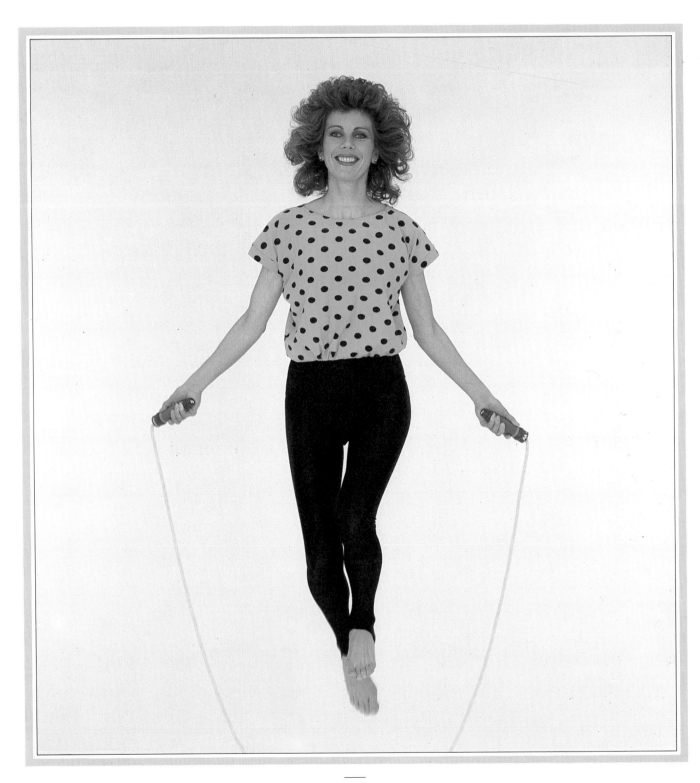

MOVEMENT *for* LIFE

All women (and men!) need to exercise, no matter what shape or size, young or old – and that includes *you*.

Where do you begin? What specific type of exercise will benefit your body – what are your capabilities and limitations? Is it enough to assume you are comparatively fit because you walk up a few stairs or stretch and bend a little as you go about your household chores? And is it true that you can achieve that long-desired perfect body shape from toning up different areas like thighs and buttocks?

First of all we must look at the importance of exercise in relation to our health. This surely is the primary reason for keeping fit. Women are particularly vulnerable to diseases such as arthritis, osteoporosis (brittle-bone disease) and heart attacks in their middle years if they have been leading a sedentary life, sitting slumped in front of the television, losing muscle tone and even bone mass.

For health insurance reasons you owe it to yourself to take care of your one and only body – your working machine. It is after all one of the

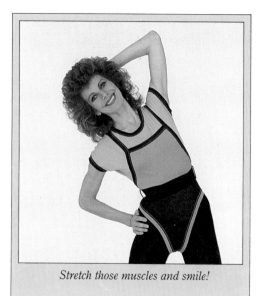
Stretch those muscles and smile!

few areas in our lives over which we have control.

A quarter of a G.P.'s surgery visits are taken up with arthritic sufferers – regular gentle exercise helps to alleviate the problem and can defer this dehabilitating disease. By the age of 50, around 44 per cent of women are overweight, compared with around 21 per cent of 20–24 year olds. Are *you* a health risk?

Before we take a look at the right fitness plan for you let's look at the physical benefits of regular exercise:

1 The biggest muscle in your body is your heart. Getting the circulation going ensures you are helping to efficiently pump gallons of blood around your body.

2 Bone-strengthening exercises like running, aerobics, skiing, swimming, brisk walking and dancing all help to maintain bone mass. Osteoporosis is a painful disease and causes broken bones and humped backs in 1 in 4 women.

3 More working days are lost in Britain through back problems than through any other single health problem. With regular exercise back and stomach muscles are strengthened, giving necessary support to the skeletal structure.

4 And for women, probably the most important physical benefit has to be the changing shape of the body. Areas of the body that are prone to flabbiness tone up – thighs, hips, stomach and arms all take on a firmer, contoured shape.

5 A fit person does not find all her energy expended on a day-to-day hectic lifestyle – there are energy reserves to enjoy a social life and leisure activities. Isn't it good to know you can sprint effortlessly for a bus, you can run up a flight of stairs without your heart thumping? That you can carry heavy bags and bend down without a twinge in the back?

PSYCHOLOGICAL BENEFITS

How many of us like our bodies, are confident with the body shape we possess? We assess and evaluate a person on an initial first impression – this includes their whole body image. If you are trying desperately to cover up your body, this will reflect not only in the way you dress but how you move. So how can exercise help?

1 Too often we only look at our faces in a mirror. Exercising in front of a mirror encourages us to take a *real* look at our bodies and get to know and control them better.

2 The sheer pleasure of enjoying the fun of exercise is reflected in our mental well-being.

3 Confidence increases. The way you move, sit and stand will show you have a greater body awareness and pride. Your body language will speak volumes about your happy state.

4 Inhibition decreases. When you are not in harmony with your body, you learn to be less tactile, less physical – learning to 'reach out' as a form of communication becomes second nature when you are used to exercising.

5 As the body tension is eased out by working out the body, muscles relax and a good sleep induced.

SPORT FOR YOU

The choice of sport is yours. But if you have any unhappy memories from being forced into team sports and cross-country runs as a school child don't try and repeat them – try something new! Evaluate what's on offer and contrast the amount of energy used against the calories consumed per hour in that activity. Look at how they compare with our normal everyday activities.

How do these sports shape-up with our Three S's – Suppleness, Stamina and Strength? When you've looked at the tables make your choice – but remember it must be enjoyable. If it doesn't achieve total fitness, make sure you use my exercise programme at least three times a week.

EXERCISE AND ENERGY				
Exercise	Calories Used (per hour)	Suppleness	Stamina	Strength
Badminton	320	●	●	●●
Cycling	350–500	●	●●●(●)	●●●(●)
Dancing				
ballet	250	●●●	●●	●●
disco	300	●●	●●●	●
Jogging	450	●	●●●	●●
Running	500–700	●	●●●(●)	●●●(●)
Skipping				
(for 15 min)	150	●	●●●	●●
Swimming				
hard	600	●●	●●●	●●●
slow	250	●●	●●	●●
Squash	600	●●	●●●	●●●
Tennis	350	●	●●	●●
Walking				
(4½ mph)	320	●	●●	●
Weight training	600–800	●●●	●●	●●●(●)

BE FRANK!

Here's a questionnaire for you to fill in. Award yourself +2 points for every 'yes' and 0 for every 'no'. Be honest with your answers and repeat the questionnaire in two months' time! And every two months try my physical tests on pages 78–80 – there are 3 tests each for the Three S's – *Strength, Suppleness and Stamina*. Always do 'The Daily Dozen' on pages 73–77 *before* attempting the tests to warm-up the body!

Your physical fitness level	Yes/No

1 Are you a non-smoker? _____

2 Do you avoid prepackaged and junk food, concentrating on fresh fruit, salads and home-cooked meals? _____

3 Do you manage to exist without sleeping pills, anti-depressants or tranquillisers? _____

4 Do you sleep well? _____

5 Do you react well to stress, remaining fairly calm and not succumbing to anxiety or tenseness? _____

6 Do you take time out for yourself at least once a day? _____

7 Are you free from muscular aches, rheumatism and back pain? _____

8 Can you bend down and touch your toes, while keeping your knees straight? _____

9 Do you have a hobby – gardening, painting, collecting – or an activity – church or women's group, political group, etc. – to which you regularly go? _____

10 Can you take easy exercise – walking or gently cycling a few miles, running up the stairs, carrying a heavy suitcase a distance – without becoming puffed or stiff? _____

11 Do you play an active sport at least once a week? _____

12 Can you do a sit-up without using your hands or anchoring your toes? _____

Your score:
0–6 Are you still alive?
7–12 You aren't too well – your lifestyle needs a radical rethink!
13–16 You are roughly average – but try reaching for higher goals.
17–20 You are doing better than average, but you need to concentrate on balancing your activity/relaxation quotient.
21–24 You *are* a healthy specimen. Keep up the good work!

What you should weigh
Firstly, your body shape will fall into one of three basic body types.

The Ectomorph frame is small with narrow shoulders and sometimes even narrower hips. It is often referred to as 'the skinny type', as there is little fat or muscle visible. Ectomorphs can look deceptively fit by virtue of their lean frame and are often agile movers.

The Mesomorph has a medium to large frame. Often the shoulders are broad and although the frame is distinctly bigger than the ectomorph, there isn't necessarily any difference in the amount of fat carried. The muscular frame lends itself to 'strength' sports and is often defined at the 'pear shape' because of the wide hips.

The Endomorph isn't necessarily large framed but is sturdily built with a large rib cage, waist and hips. Unfortunately fat is to often accumulated in these areas. Speed sports are not their favourite but swimming is ideal.

Having decided upon your frame category, check your height and ideal weight with the chart.

Don't become obsessive about weighing yourself – I very rarely step on the scales. The only way you can have a reasonably fair assessment of weight loss if you are trying to lose weight is to weigh yourself once a week, on the same scales, at the same time of the day and preferably with no clothes on! Better still, an honest appraisal of yourself standing naked in front of a full-length mirror will help you come to terms with the frame you have and everything you are aiming to achieve.

WHAT SHOULD YOU WEIGH?

Height ft in	Small frame st lb (lbs)			Medium frame st lb (lbs)			Large frame st lb (lbs)		
4 8	6	8	(92)	6	13	(97)	7	8	(106)
4 9	6	10	(94)	7	1	(99)	7	11	(109)
4 10	7	0	(98)	7	7	(105)	8	2	(114)
4 11	7	3	(101)	7	11	(109)	8	5	(117)
5 0	7	6	(104)	8	0	(112)	8	8	(120)
5 1	7	9	(107)	8	2	(114)	8	11	(123)
5 2	7	12	(110)	8	5	(117)	9	0	(126)
5 3	8	1	(113)	8	8	(120)	9	3	(129)
5 4	8	4	(116)	8	12	(124)	9	7	(133)
5 5	8	7	(119)	9	1	(127)	9	11	(137)
5 6	8	11	(123)	9	5	(131)	10	1	(141)
5 7	9	1	(127)	9	9	(135)	10	4	(144)
5 8	9	5	(131)	9	13	(139)	10	8	(148)
5 9	9	8	(134)	10	3	(143)	10	12	(152)
5 10	10	0	(140)	10	6	(146)	11	1	(155)
5 11	10	4	(144)	10	10	(150)	11	6	(160)
6 0	10	8	(148)	10	13	(153)	11	11	(165)

To help determine your frame size, measure your wrists and ankles at their narrowest points.

For wrists, 5½in (14cm) or less is small, 6in (15cm) is medium, and 6½in (16.5cm) or more is large.

The measurements for ankles are 8in (20cm), 8½in (21.5cm) and 9in (23cm) respectively.

BEGINNING AT THE BEGINNING – FIRST STEPS

With this exercise plan you will notice an enormous improvement in your stamina, suppleness and strength after just seven days. Before you attempt the programme, check the reminders so that you can get the maximum possible results.

1 Wear loose, comfortable clothing if you are not exercising in leotards and tights.

2 Bare feet are best.

3 Don't eat a heavy meal for at least two hours before you exercise.

4 Exercise at least 3 times a week at a time that suits you best.

5 If you are not feeling well, conserve your energy for getting better. Leave your exercise programme until you have recovered.

6 Always STOP if anything hurts – listen to your body.

7 Never strain. You will damage your body if you try and over-achieve.

8 The key to total fitness is to build up gradually – find your own level to begin with. As you improve, increase the number of times you do each exercise.

* If you are in any doubt as the whether you should be attempting these exercises, consult your doctor – particularly if you suffer from a heart condition, a serious weight problem, varicose veins or an asthmatic illness.

These exercises can be done to a strong rhythm, so choose a record that you will enjoy working out to. If necessary half-time your exercises to the music beat – slow exercises not only minimise the risk of incorrect positioning but take more effort to sustain!

THE DAILY DOZEN

Look how easy it is – these 12 exercises will keep you feeling young and lithe, full of vitality and the satisfaction of knowing that you are taking care of your body. Taking responsibility for your joints and limbs – knowing that it can only enhance and better the quality of your life – *is* this easy! If you cannot do them daily, try and make sure you do them every alternate day. But I am sure you will find the time – 10 minutes! – so do them daily because you will miss them if you don't. Whether you are 20 or 80 years-old you can take care of yourself.

You know your own body, its capabilities and limitations, I do not want to specify the number of times you should attempt each exercise. It is possible that you can achieve 6 of each exercise, for some 12. Do what is comfortable and keep a note of how many you can do. You might like to count your way through out loud, some people like to sing and, if you do have a full-length mirror you can exercise in front of, then watch yourself. Join me every day at the time that suits you best. The first days may be hard, but you'll soon get into it.

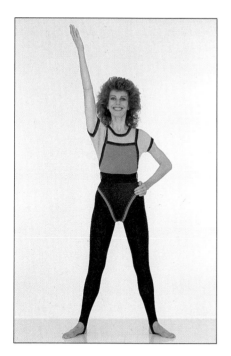

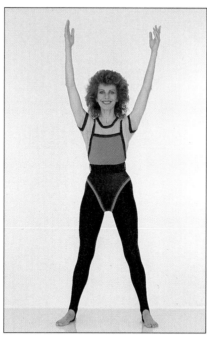

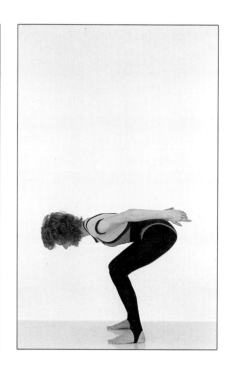

1 Stand with your legs and feet a comfortable distance apart. Place both hands on your hips. Raise your right arm up in the air close to your head, then place back on your hip, repeat with your left arm.

2a Ski down those slopes: With toes facing the front, raise both arms above your head. Bend your legs at the knees and swoop your arms down and behind your bottom, in one movement.

2b Swing your arms back up through this action, returning to a standing, upright position. As you stand, pull in the tummy and pull up, out of the hips. Do *not* arch the back.

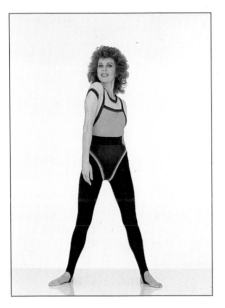

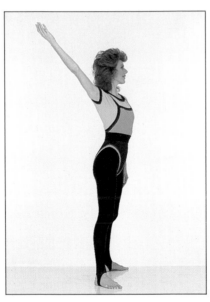

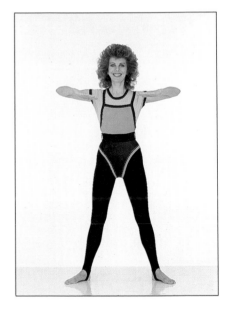

3 Loosely circle your right shoulder forward, up, and around. Don't strain the neck. Relax those shoulders as you repeat the exercise with your left shoulder.

4 Slowly circle your right arm forward, then up and behind. Bring it down slowly . . . and round back up. Do this all in one continuous flowing motion.

5 Bend your arms in front of you at chest height, shoulders down.

Ease the elbows back, working the upper arms. You will only be able to do so if you keep them raised. Flow the movement.

6 Bend both legs. Clasp your arms just above the wrists. Turning from the waist, twist to your right side. Come back to your centre and repeat the action to your left.

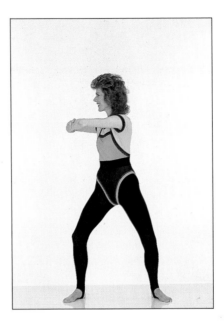

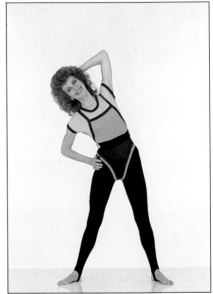

7 (All waist exercises should be done without any strain or jerking. Always remember, before you lean to your side, to pull out of the hips. This works your waist properly. Think 'Pull up to go over!')

Raise your left arm, bending to place your left hand lightly behind your head. Lean to your right side, gently easing the waist into that position. Return to start. Now lightly place your right hand behind your head and lean to your left side.

8 For a greater stretch, raise your left arm up above your head and lean to your right side.

Raise your right arm up and lean to your left side.

(Notice how, in both these waist exercises, the weight is also supported by the non-working arm with the hand placed at the top of the thigh.)

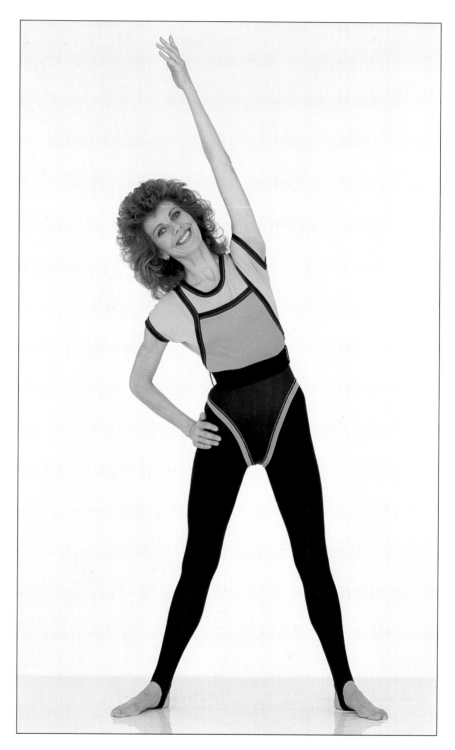

9 Turning out from the top of the thighs, bend both legs. Keep your feet flat on the floor and deeply bend. Don't let your feet roll inwards and keep your knees over the toes!

Now straighten up, using the strength in your thighs.

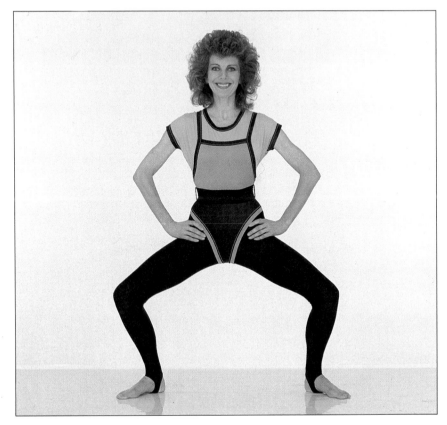

10 Raise your right knee up straight in front of you, hold for a moment, then lower. Raise your left knee and hold. Keep alternating legs.

11 Lightly clasp your hands together behind the back of your head. Raise your knee to chest height. Lean forward and place your opposite elbow on the knee to lightly touch it. As your left elbow touches your right knee turn to see your right side. Reverse as your right elbow touches your left knee, turning to see the left side. Alternate legs.

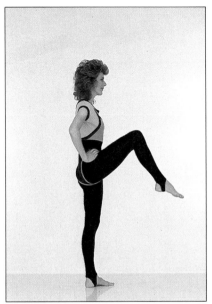

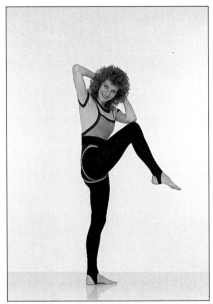

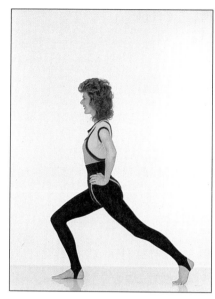

12 Take it away and lunge! Face your right side. Bend your right leg and, keeping your left leg straight, extend it behind you with your toes curled. Feel the stretch in that position – your standing leg will get lower as you obtain greater thigh strength.

Now face your left side. Bend your left leg in front and extend the right leg.

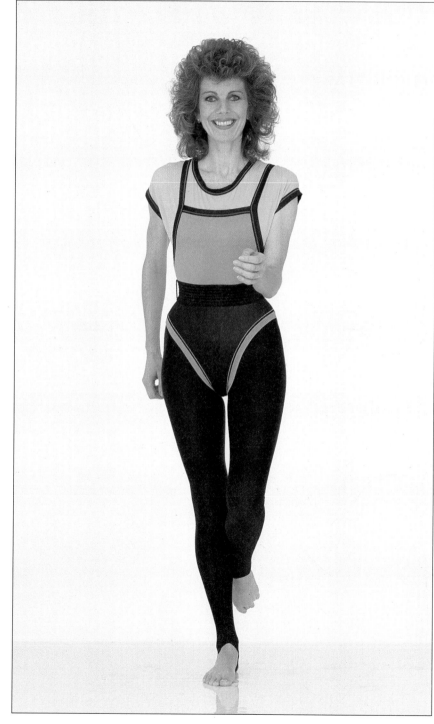

Now you've worked through these 12 exercises, lightly jog for a few seconds and remember to jog where you can, whether it's going for a bus or running up the stairs. Your daily dozen exercises don't just stop here!

TESTS FOR THE THREE S'S

Test yourself on these three sets of exercises every two months – after you have completed the questionnaire and warmed up with The Daily Dozen. Don't push yourself on these exercises either; work your way into Stamina – after all,

that's what it means: staying power. A positive attitude is an important asset when it comes to maintaining a workout regime, and that comes with knowing that you are not pitting yourself against the impossible.

STRENGTH
– so your body can exert its maximum force

TUMMY SIT UPS
Lay on the floor with legs and knees apart and drawn up, hands *lightly* clasped behind the head. Working through a curved spine, can you do a dozen sit ups?

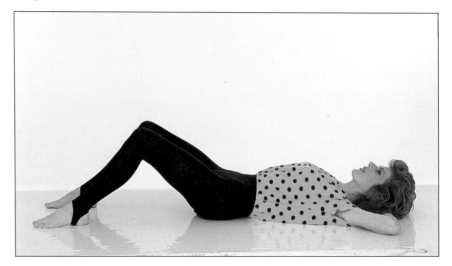

PRESS UPS
This is great for biceps and shoulders. Lie face downwards, palms on the floor at shoulder level, toes pointed. Balance on the balls of your feet. Straighten your arms, raising your body in a straight line, and lower. Can you repeat this 3 times?

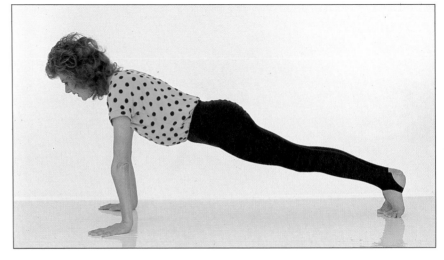

THIGH STRENGTH

Kneel on one leg. Raise the toes of the back leg and – without the toes touching back on the floor – stand up, using the thigh strength of the front leg. Now change legs – can you do this effortlessly or do you find you have one leg stronger than the other?

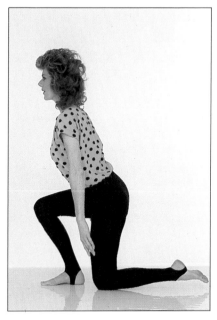
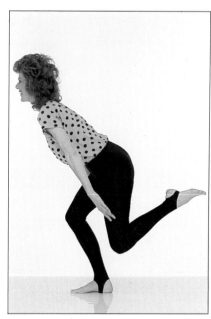

SUPPLENESS
– for freedom of movement

WAIST FLEXIBILITY

Stand with your legs and feet a comfortable distance apart. Lightly clasp your hands behind your head, elbows out to the sides. Lean to your right side – can your elbow touch your thigh? Come up and repeat to your left side.

SHOULDERS

Stand straight and lift your right arm above your head. Bend your right elbow, dropping your forearm behind your back and see if you can clasp the fingers of your right hand with those of your left. Now try the other side – notice how one side seems to be more flexible!

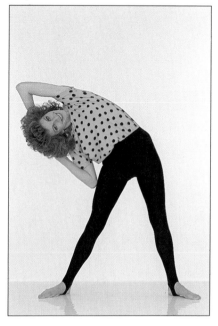
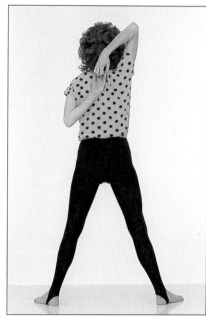

TORSO

Sit on the floor, legs forming a 'V' a comfortable distance apart. Lightly clasp your hands behind your head. Roll slightly back on your hips and, turning to face your right knee, aim to bring your left elbow to your right knee. Return to sitting position and try to touch your left knee with your right elbow.

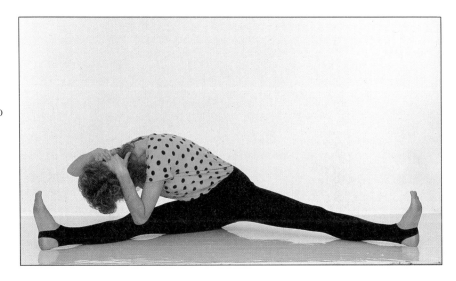

STAMINA
– to give you staying power

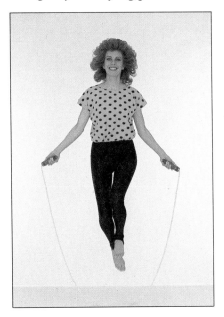

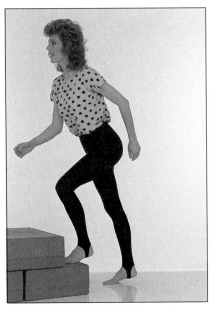

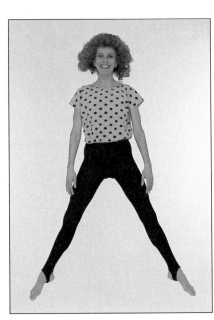

1 Without bending or leaning forward, skip rhythmically fast for 60 seconds. Can you repeat it?

2 Run up two dozen stairs or more without being breathless at the top.

3 Can you do 12 Star Jumps and hold a conversation afterwards – without puffing and panting!

EXERCISES
for SPECIFIC AREAS

We all have a problem area that we would like to change. *We* consider it a problem, though invariably others don't understand what on earth we are talking about. You can take comfort that you are not alone. I have met nobody that is wholly satisfied with the body God gave them – but this is the body you've got so you'd better make the best of it. Not only do we need to strengthen up the entire body to keep it in good working order but there are certain areas that need extra exercise to give the area more definition; areas that accumulate unwanted flab. 'The Seven Great Areas of Women' are all accounted for here and, of course, as the years go by the number seems to increase!

Men have different physiological problems, chief among them weight gain caused by lack of exercise. I am often bemused by the men who criticize a woman's shape when they are quite clearly looking down on their own unsightly 'pregnant'-looking stomachs. It can be very demoralising for a man to find that his partner, though somewhat advancing in age, is diminish-

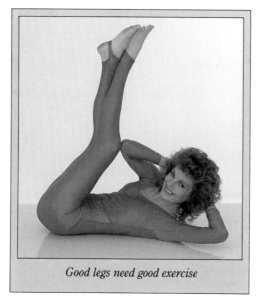

Good legs need good exercise

ing in size. A thoroughly toned-up body with sleek limbs, a sparkle in the eye and a lack of double chins can keep you looking mischievously young when you're the wrong side of 40!

Can you admire or respect a successful businessman at the age of fifty who has accumulated wealth, yet lost his health while doctors warn 'Lose at least 5 stones and stop drinking or you will be dead before your next birthday'? Success cannot be measured in material terms when such blinding indulgence overrides the enjoyment of physical well-being. But it is we women who can sport a trim ankle and a shapely calf muscle, whether the hemlines are fashionably raised or fallen, so included here are some exercises for the ankles and calves. Our feet and legs deserve greater attention than we give because of the abuse they tolerate every day. For at least fifteen hours a day they get us from A to B and take our body weight. Invariably our toes are unnaturally cramped into odd-shaped shoes and the feet raised because we choose to teeter around in high heels!

BEAUTIFUL LEGS *(don't forget the bottom!)*

Before you attempt some – if not all – of these exercises, you must warm-up first with 'The Daily Dozen'. Then, work on your calves and ankles so you are ready to concentrate on more advanced leg exercises.

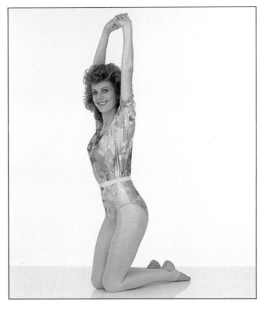

1 Kneel, feet and legs together, arms stretched above your head, hands clasped together. Lower yourself back to your heels, but don't sit back on them. Rise straight back up through the strength in your thighs. You can also circle your hips, swooping down to your heels as you go round and come up to the other side!

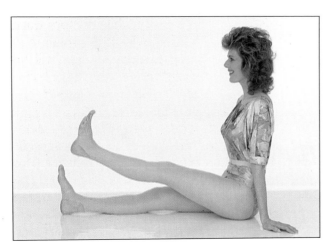

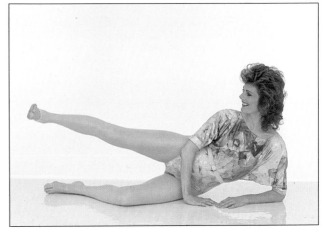

2 Sit on the floor, both legs outstretched in front, hands placed either side of you. Flex your feet so your toes are pointed to the ceiling. Raise and lower your left leg, not too high in a fast, continuous movement. Pull up your leg muscles and feel how solid that left thigh is becoming! Shake out your left leg and repeat the exercise with your right.

3 Lie on your left side, supported by your left arm, the right arm placed in front, your left leg bent underneath. Raise your right leg, flexing the foot so that your toes are pointed toward the front. Raise and lower your right leg in fast, continuous movements. When your outer thigh starts to shake or hurt, stop. You have achieved the maximum effect with this exercise.

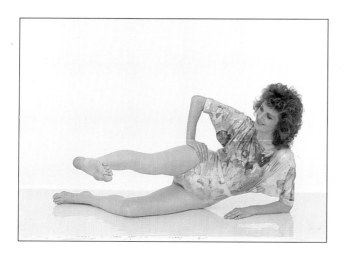

4a Lying on your side, place your right hand at the top of your right thigh. Keep your foot flexed and start slowly circling your right leg, at the same time bringing it up in the air.

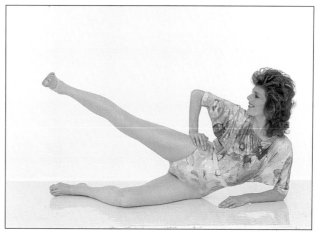

4b Carry it to the side and around. Keep the circle flowing – you might only achieve 4 times to begin with.

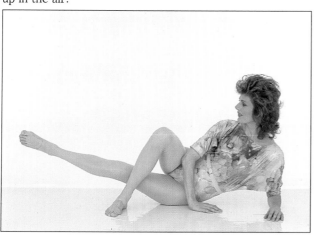

5 Lying on your side, cross your right leg over your left leg. Raise and straighten your left leg, pointing the toes up and down.

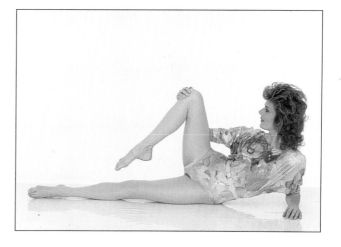

6 Lying on your side, bend your right leg and support it just below the knee with your hand. Ease the thigh back towards your chest.

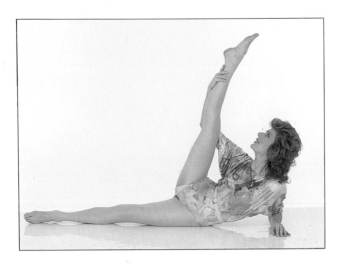

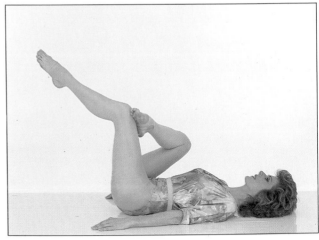

7 Lying on your side, lift your straight leg high in the air, supporting it at the back of the ankle or at the calf muscle. Your leg might not be able to go back very far to start with.

8 Lie flat on your back and loosen up your hip. Bend your left leg and bend your right leg out to the side. Hook your right toes or ankle above your left knee and gently ease your left leg back in small slow movements. This will loosen up your right hip.

Now repeat exercises 3 – 8 working the opposite leg.

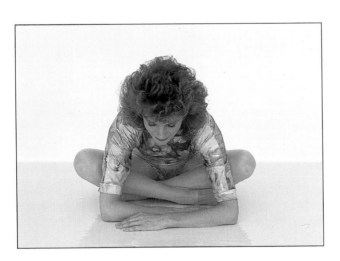

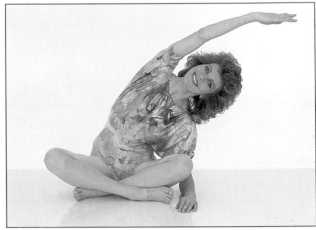

9 Sit cross-legged on the floor and ease forward out of the hips. It takes a good deal of suppleness to be able to get both your elbows onto the ground – you might only get your hands flat on the floor to begin with.

10 Continue to sit cross-legged. Turn to your right side and attempt to touch the floor with your elbow, and then turn and try your left. Now stretch your right arm over your head, balancing on your left arm which is by your side. Reach over and then change sides.

11 Sit with your feet and legs apart – do not over-extend the distance – it defeats the purpose of the exercise and you will find you won't be able to walk properly the next day! Body alignment is very important with this exercise.

Turn to face your right leg so that your torso is in line with your right leg. Place your hands either side of your leg and gently ease forward. Now repeat the exercise with your torso directly in line with your left leg.

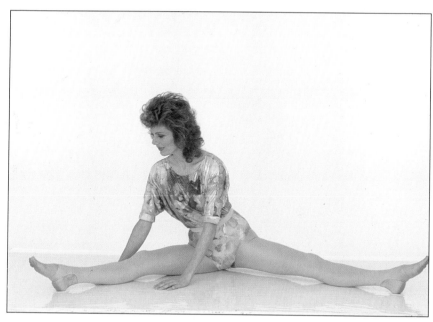

12 Now reach over your right leg with your left arm stretched right over your head. Repeat this position over your left leg with your right arm over your head.

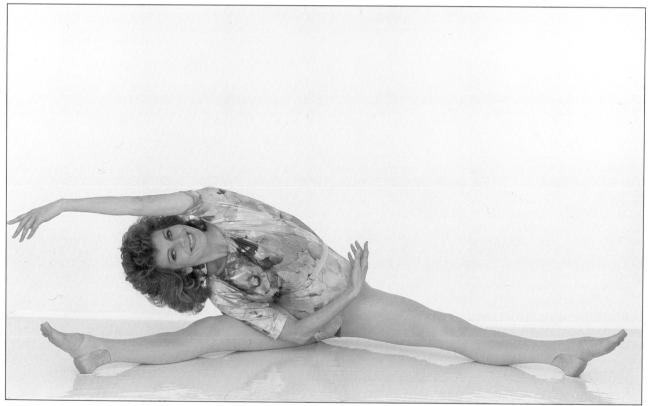

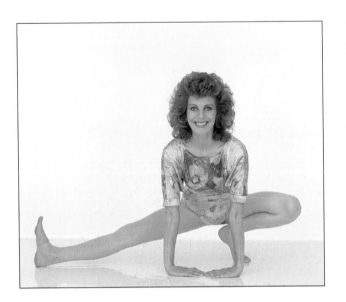

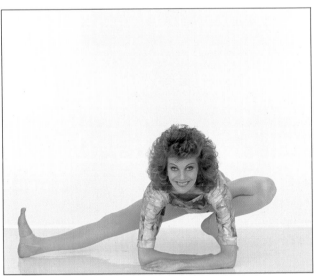

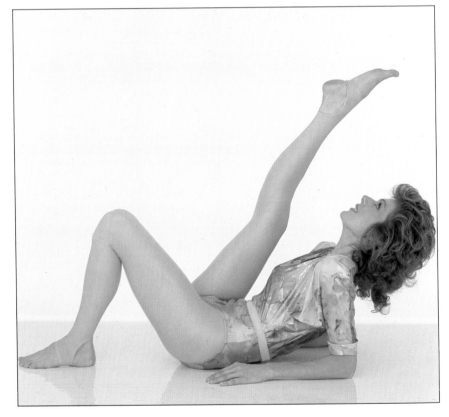

13 Crouch and extend your right leg out to the side with your foot flexed. Keep your left knee turned out to the side, and place your hands through the gap in front of you on the floor. Gently ease into this position and repeat with your left leg out to the side.

14 Hold the above position. See if you can ease forward sufficiently to relax your elbows onto the ground. If the insides of the thighs are stretching, then you are attempting this exercise too early in your fitness programme.

15 Lie back on your elbows and enjoy the freedom of a high kick! Bend your left leg to support your back and kick your right leg straight up and down. To help control the muscles, including the tummy, you can keep the leg 2 inches off the floor as the leg comes down. Bend your right leg and practise kicking your left leg. Keep a score on these exercises.

ARMS AND SHOULDERS

One of the areas that shows the first signs of body ageing is the upper arms – they can become thick and flabby and as a result shapeless. These exercises will firm up these vulnerable areas and if this routine is done daily then you will not only quickly see a noticeable difference, but feel the strength and power in your arms as you go about your everyday business. Hands and arms are like our feet and legs, constantly in demand! But do not forget the shoulders. Not only are they vital to our posture, they help keep the torso flexible. If you stoop or are round-shouldered these shoulder movements will help to rectify this problem area for you. Very often teenager girls become physically inhibited. As their breasts grow, they round their shoulders. Do encourage them to do this exercise routine too.

Tension – and we know it well! – collects around the neck and shoulder area, so it is important that you try and relax the muscles in that region before you start any exercise programme. 'Shake out' the shoulders and arms before you begin. I personally never start my exercise routine with the head and neck exercises in which you look from side to side and circle the head round. If you are feeling tense, you can be totally unaware of *how* tense. You may begin doing these exercises 'cold', causing further damage to your neck and shoulders.

Here is a very useful tip. If you are feeling nervous before an interview, a party or just need a confidence booster, then run through these specific area exercises. Not only will they relax you, but you will 'square up to the world', with your shoulders back, with the correct carriage of your head, and a poise that proudly says 'This Is Me.'

At first you will feel a general ache in the arms and shoulders from attempting some of these exercises. When your arms become too heavy to hold either out to your sides or above your head, or they start trembling, it is time to stop. Keep a regular check on your score – you might only achieve 8 repetitions of one exercise, 4 of another and 20 of a different exercise!

Stand comfortably, feet and legs a little apart. Should at any time the muscles feel fatigued, 'shake out' the arms. Relax until they feel ready to continue.

> Do remember that strong arm muscles and shoulders will help protect the back. If you are ever carrying heavy loads, break up the load into a number of cases or boxes at approximately the same weight. If you have heavy equipment to transport, don't just sling it over one shoulder; try to equalize the load.

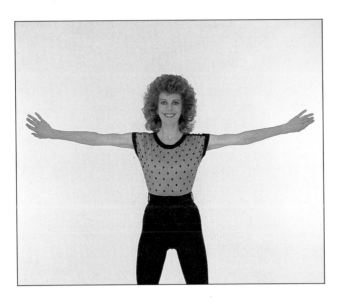

1 Raise both arms out to your sides. Rhythmically twist both arms over and back, over and back.

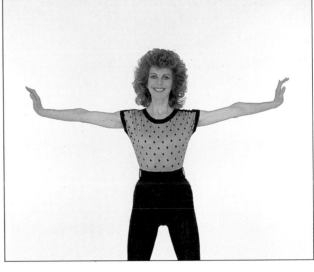

2 Stretch your arms out to the sides, flex both hands, and draw small, quick tight circles round one way. Complete your attempted number and circle the other way. Make sure that your arms are straight.

3a Still with your arms straight, flex your hands and cross your arms low in front of you, hands together. Continuing to keep your arms crossed tightly over each other, raise them to chest height.

3b Raise your crossed arms above your head. Follow through the exercise by lowering them. The tighter you keep the movement the more beneficial the exercise.

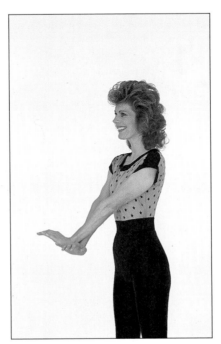

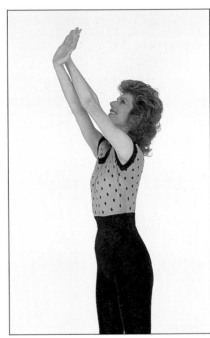

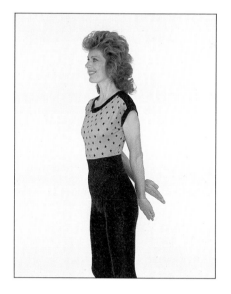

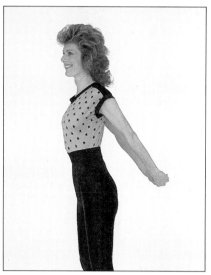

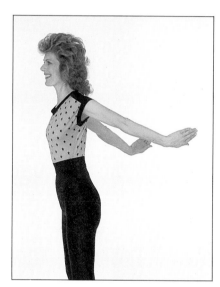

4 Stand tall. Repeat the criss-crossing of the arms, but this time low behind your back. The fingers and hands should be pointing downwards in this exercise.

5 Clasp your hands behind your back – it is sometimes easier if one hand grasps the thumb of the other hand. Slowly raise and lower your arms. See how high you can raise them.

6 Raise your arms high behind you, but keep your shoulders down. Now raise the arms in small repetitive movements. Don't allow your head to poke forward.

7 Let both arms fall forward so that the backs of the wrists are just touching.
   Slowly take both arms back behind you, until the fingertips are touching. Feel the muscles on the inside of the upper arm working.

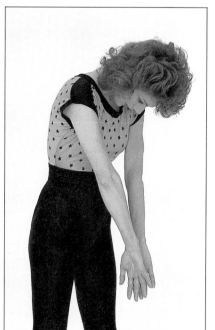

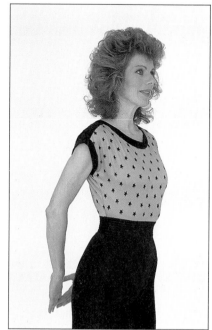

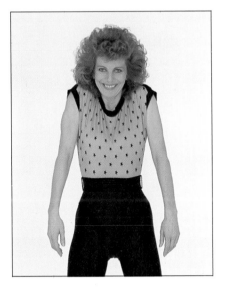

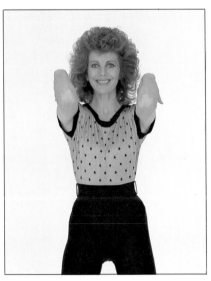

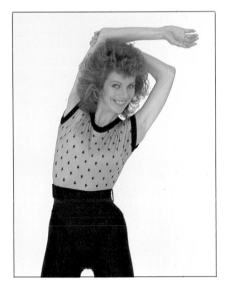

8 Lightly shrug both shoulders, bringing them up to your ears, then dropping them down.

9 Place the fingertips of both hands on your shoulders, bending your arms at the elbow. Guide your elbows through a series of small circles.

10 Bend your left arm over your head, holding it below the left elbow with your right hand. This will loosen up your left shoulder as you gently ease your left arm further over your head. Bring your supported arm back to level. This is a great exercise for flexibility.

Repeat the same exercise, holding your right arm below the elbow by stretching over your left arm.

11 Punch away those troubles. Bend your legs a little and punch each arm in front of you, changing arms with each punch. The effort should come from behind the shoulder. Think of all the things you want to hit! This will help you punch realistically hard. It certainly relieves any tension around the shoulders!

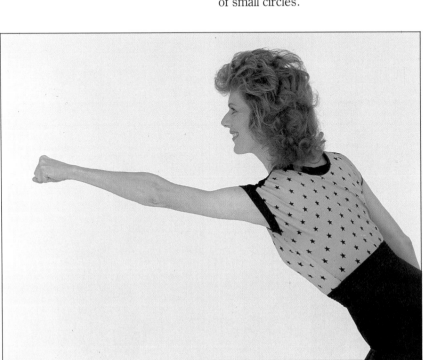

BACK EXERCISES

The back is a delicate instrument, and so finely tuned that nearly everyone of us at some time has experienced some sort of back problem. Twisting the small of the back or slipping a disc are common complaints, while pains are suffered by millions of people everyday. Incorrect body balance, a sudden wrenching as you swivel round can, in a split second, cause you back problems for the rest of your life. Here are six back exercises which will help strengthen the back muscles and stretch the spine. Select those exercises which you are capable of doing without suffering any pain. You know your body better than any exercise teacher or doctor; if any of these exercises causes any doubt in your mind as to whether you should be doing them, avoid having a go until you have consulted a doctor.

We will start with my favourite stretching exercise. It can also be done sitting in a chair. Why not get used to doing this stretch throughout the day – especially if you have been sitting in the same position for any length of time? Notice how the legs are bent – good training for everyday tasks. Whenever you pick up a heavy load, bend both legs. The thighs should take the main weight of the load.

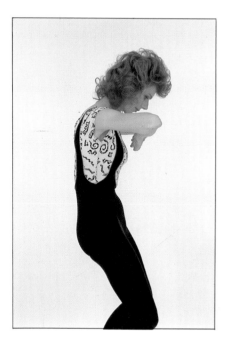

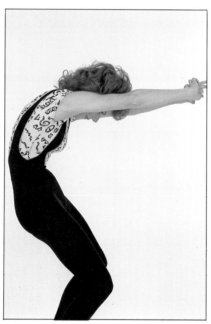

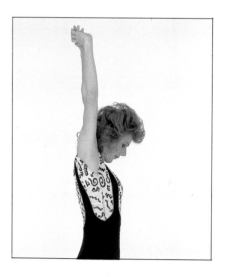

1c Now raise your arms above your head, straightening the legs and your spine. This is one continuous flowing movement. Hold that stretch, pulling and elongating the spine from the very base out of the hips, chin to chest. Part your hands, bring the arms out to your sides, and lower. Repeat.

1a With the back of the hands facing inwards, place one hand over the other. Bend the arms at the elbows.

1b Push away the arms, forcing the hands out. As they straighten, curve the spine and pull in the tummy, as if you have just received a blow.

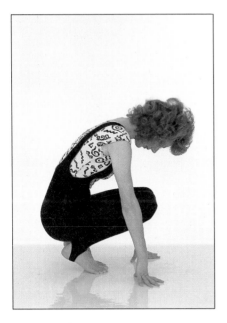

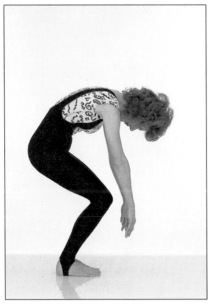

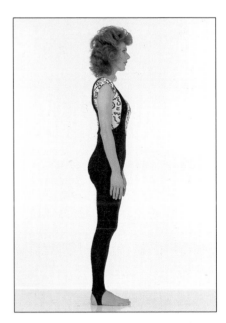

2a For correct posture crouch on the floor, knees and feet together, heels off the floor.

2b Slowly rise up, lowering your heels to the floor. Keep arms hanging, head down and neck and shoulders relaxed.

2c Slowly come up into the final standing position. Arms by your sides, shoulders relaxed, head correctly positioned as you look straight in front. Do *not* arch the back with your bottom sticking out.

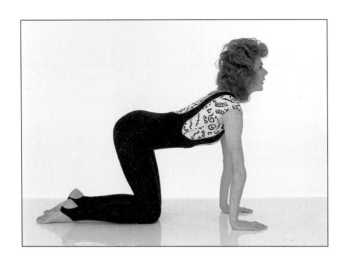

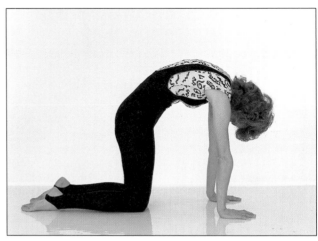

3a Kneel on all fours, feet and knees apart. Arch your back as high as you can and drop your head.

3b Reverse your back position by pushing the spine downwards in a curve. Stick your bottom up.

4a Kneel on your left knee, head down. Swing your right knee toward the front, so that it almost touches your forehead.

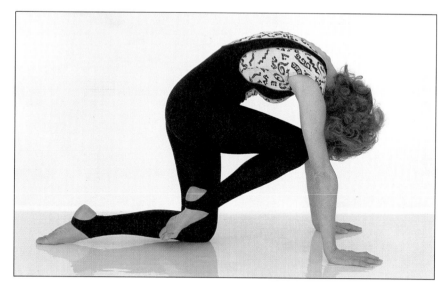

4b Bring the right leg back, knee bent, then extend it straight out behind you as high as you can. Keep hips facing forward, allowing no twisting. Do not rush the swing forward and back – the movements should swing into each other. Repeat the exercise, this time kneeling on your right knee, and exercising the left leg.

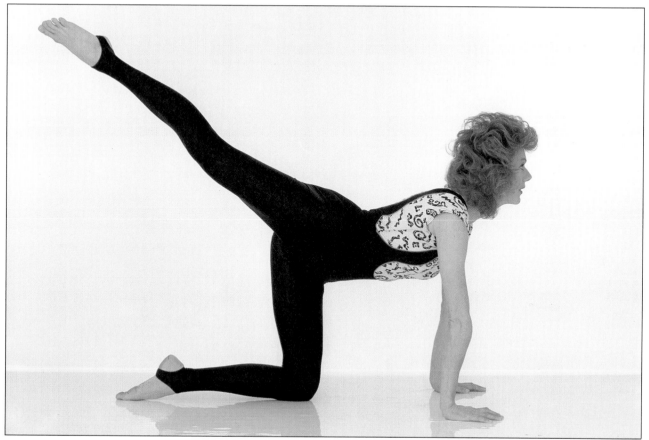

5 Bend your arms in front of you, so that you are resting some of your weight on your elbows. Raise your right leg straight and high up behind you – with no hip twisting. Repeat using the left leg.

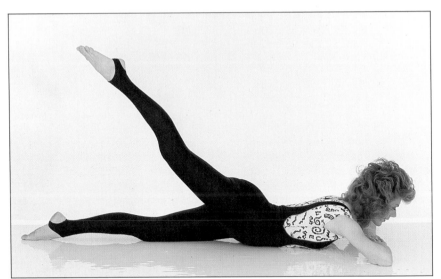

6 Lie flat on the floor, arms and legs extended. Imagine you are flying through the air – raise both arms and legs simultaneously. Hold this position for a slow count of 4 and lower.

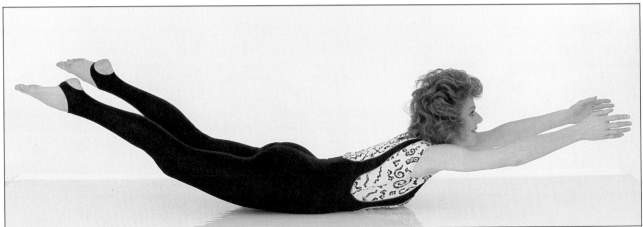

7 To relax the back, kneel and place your arms either side of your body on the floor, rest your forehead on the floor. Stay in this position for some time, then slowly sit up through a curved spine – a great way to relax!

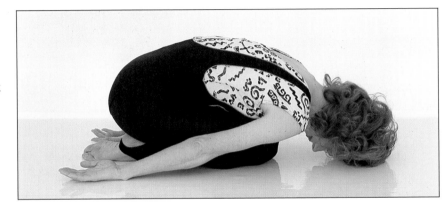

TUMMY EXERCISES

These tummy exercises are particularly suitable for anyone who has had a baby or a hysterectomy. They are very gentle and, as the muscles regain their strength, you can increase the number of times they are repeated. Once they are manageable then the tummy strengthener exercises can be attempted.

Most of these exercises are done with the aid of the hands to support the weakened muscles. But always work on the proviso that you will stop if the tummy either twinges or aches.

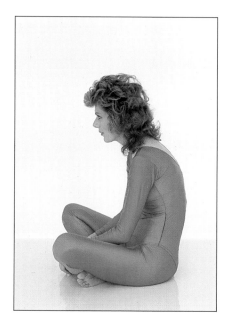

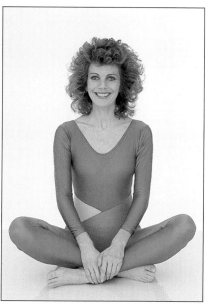

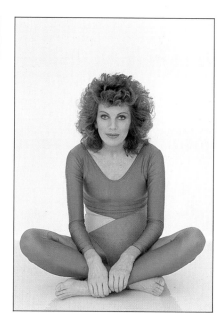

1 Sit cross-legged on the floor or bed and slump – easily done! Now the stomach muscles are completely relaxed.

2 Sit up straight, and hold on lightly to your ankles if you so wish. Pull in the tummy muscles and hold that position. This is also good for posture.

3 Sit cross-legged and slump again – notice just how ungainly and bad for the body this is. But look around you and see how many people sit just like this!

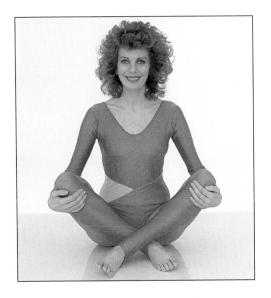

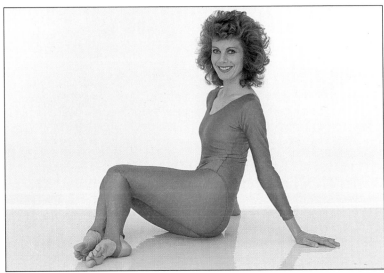

4 Pull yourself up straight again, sitting up as tall as you can. Pull the tummy muscles in hard, while lightly holding on just below your knees.

5a Twist and turn across your body. Place your hands to your sides, draw up your knees toward your chin and, keeping your knees together, roll on your bottom, allowing your knees to roll to your right side. They might nowhere near touch the ground!

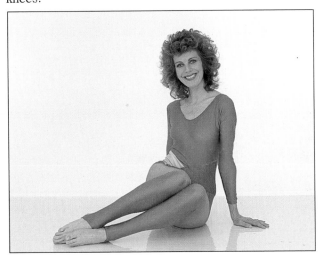

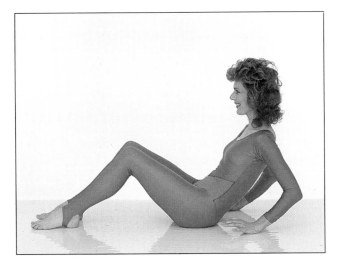

5b Bring your knees back up to the centre and let them roll across your body over to your left side. Repeat the roll on your right side.

6 Sit on the ground. Place your hands behind you, draw up your feet, keeping your knees a comfortable distance apart, and gently rock backwards and forwards. Make sure you lean back through a *curved* spine and rock off the heel of your hands for added support.

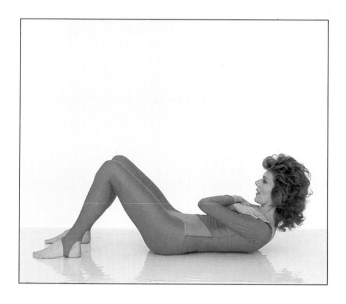

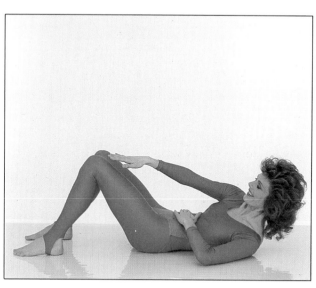

7 Lie down. Keep your knees drawn up and fold your arms across your chest. Raise your head and shoulders, breathing out. Lie down again. Repeat.

8a Place your hands on your tummy. Raise your head and shoulders, placing your right fingertips on your left knee. Lie flat down again.

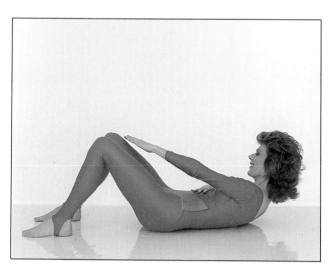

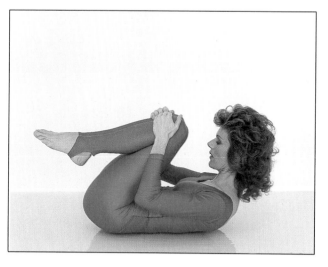

8b Repeat the exercise, but place your left fingertips onto your right knee.

9 Raise your head and shoulders. Hug in both knees to your chest. Hold for a slow count of 4. Lie back down again, placing your legs back on the floor, knees bent.

Once you can achieve all these exercises with several repetitions and with absolutely no discomfort, then attempt the tummy strengtheners and flatteners.

MORE STOMACH STRENGTHENERS AND FLATTENERS

Go for it! Where do you begin? SLOWLY.

Some of these exercises are difficult to achieve and as you look at them, some of them could be way beyond your grasp – for the moment. Select the ones you can achieve before graduating to the more strenuous ones. A flat tummy and strong working centre muscles can take years to build up – and a very short time to render them null and void! It can be the birth of a baby, a hysterectomy, or a lazy, sedentary lifestyle with an unhealthy indulgence in all

the wrong type of foods that cause the spare tyre and those extra pounds of wobbling fat.

If you are now feeling completely at ease with Stage 1 of the tummy exercises and you have mastered at least 8 repeats of each exercise then start working on Stage 2 – not only will you look good, you will take the strain off your back.

You do not have to continue with stage 1 exercises if you find no further need of them or you want to concentrate fully on these harder exercises!

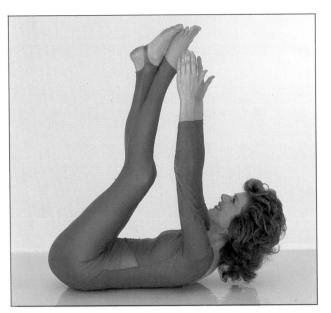

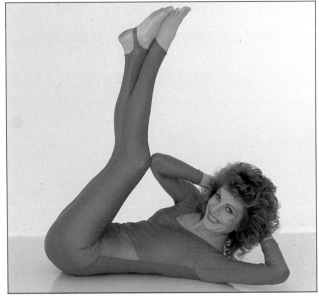

10 Lie flat on your back. Raise both legs in the air, crossing them at the ankles; bend your legs a little. Raise your head and keep reaching for your ankles – maybe even past them for your toes. Do not drop your head back onto the floor at all. If you can achieve 20 reaches you are doing well!

11 Still with your legs crossed in the air, lightly clasp your hands behind your head. Sit up a little and touch your right elbow onto your left knee and then your left elbow onto your right knee. Keep a nice rhythmic swing to this. How many can you do?

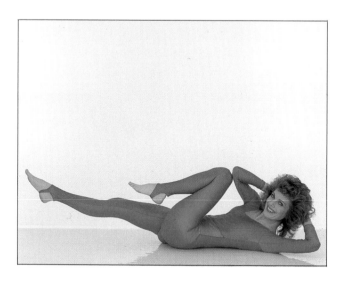

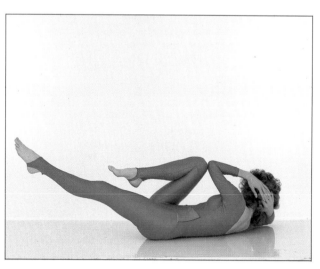

11a Bend your left knee, extend your right leg and touch your right elbow onto your left knee.

11b Change legs. Extend your left leg and bend your right. Touch your right leg with your left elbow. It is a strange way to cycle!

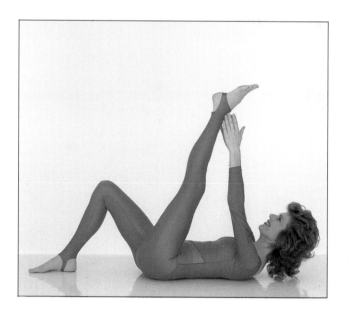

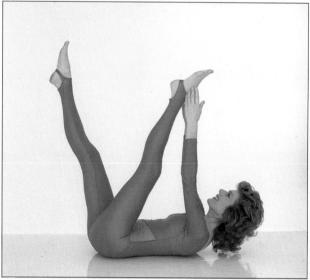

12 Bend your right leg and raise your left leg high in the air. Raise your head. With a small rocking movement, reach for the ankle of your left foot – lifting up and back off your shoulders. Repeat the exercise with your right leg in the air and your left leg bent on the floor. Not easy this!

13 The same exercise can be done with both legs in the air – but you do need excellent stomach control in order to do this. Make sure the curve of your spine is pressed into the floor.

14a Rowing time – but without the machine! Balance on your bottom, knees together, feet off the ground, arms bent holding the 'oars'.

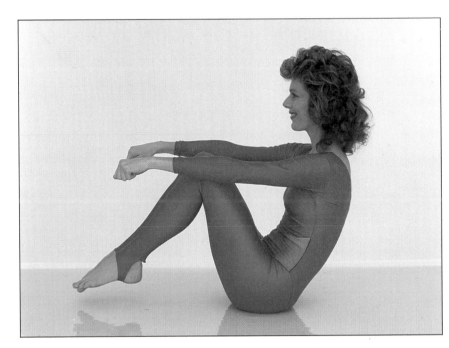

14b Exhale as you lean back – not too far – through a curved spine. Reach out with the arms. Both movements should be combined and executed quickly. Do not hold the leaning back position.

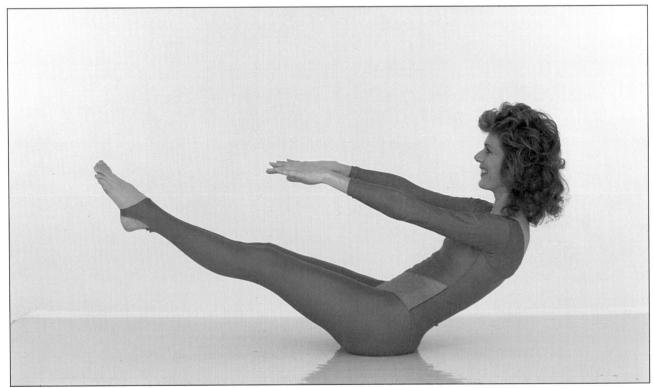

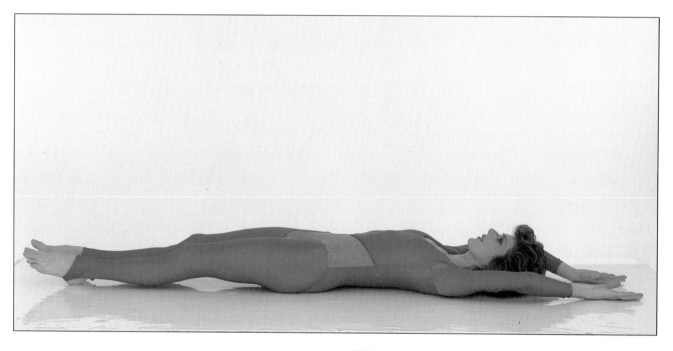

15a The Jack Knife
The ultimate stomach floor exercise! Lie flat, arms outstretched above the head, feet and legs together. Do not hollow the back.

15b In one single movement, raise both the torso and the legs – up through a curved spine to a sitting position, grasping the ankles. Sit in triumph, then lie flat back down again and repeat!

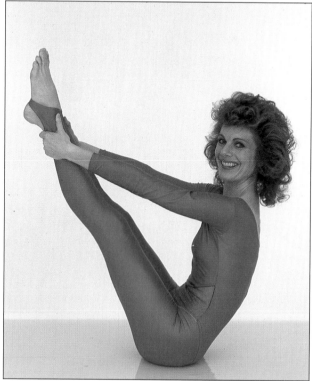

WAIST EXERCISES

The waist is one of the most rewarding areas to see visual improvement upon quickly, by means of regular, concentrated waist exercises. If you consistently – and by that I mean once or twice daily – follow this waist plan you will feel and see a definite toning up of the whole line. Your middle area will become firmer and your posture will improve dramatically.

But the exercises must be done correctly. Before you start any waist exercise, check that you are centred, leaning neither forwards nor backwards; that your legs and feet are a comfortable distance apart and your bottom tucked under. Always in your mind's eye see yourself as you stretch either upwards or towards your sides, 'growing' at least two inches out of the hip. You need to pull out of your hips first before you start any waist exercise. Now let's 'waist away'!

Attempt each exercise a minimum of 4 times to begin with. Gradually increase the number each time you do this set of exercises. *Never* 'yank' to your sides or as you reach up – the movement should be gentle and minimal. If you feel any twinge of pain in the back, readjust your position. It is possible that your body is incorrectly aligned. If there is further pain, do not do that particular exercise.

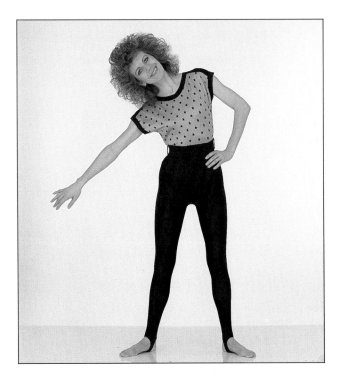

1 Place your left hand on your hip. Reach down to your right with your right arm.

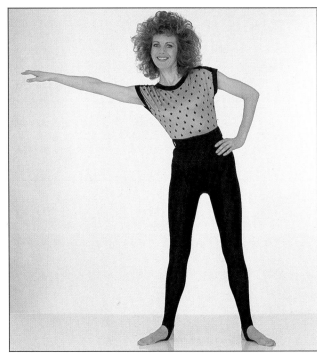

2 Take your right arm out to the side, stretching out with a gentle 'rocking' motion as if you were trying to reach something.

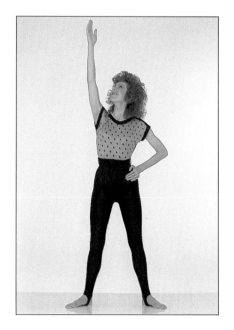

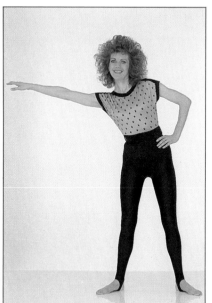

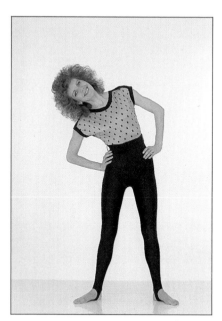

3 Repeat that same action with your right arm raised above your head. Feel the stretch out of your right hip.

4 Return your right arm to the side and reach out again.

Repeat exercises 1–4 with your left arm.

5 Place both hands on your hips and lean to your right side. With a small movement, rock to your right side for as many times as is comfortable. Repeat to your left.

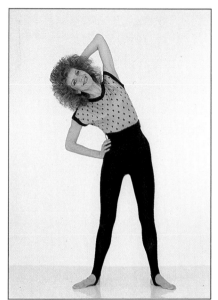

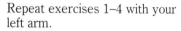

6 Place your left hand behind your head and lean to your right side. Keep your elbow pointed up to the ceiling to stretch correctly – notice how the waist is quite clearly defined with this exercise. Now reverse it – right hand behind your head, left hand on hip and lean to your left.

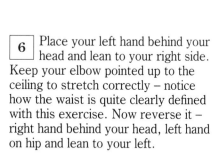

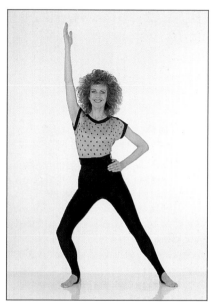

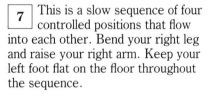

7 This is a slow sequence of four controlled positions that flow into each other. Bend your right leg and raise your right arm. Keep your left foot flat on the floor throughout the sequence.

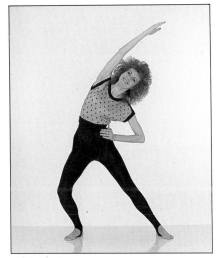

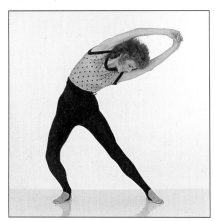

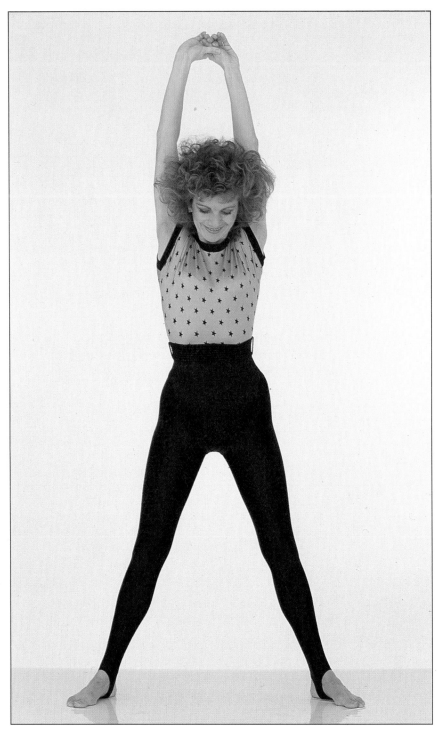

8 Reach over to your left side, curving from your right arm.

9 Holding that position join your left hand and arm, clasp hands.

10 Pull back via your arms to the centre. Straighten both legs and stretch right out of your hips; straighten the spine and let your chin fall to your chest. Lower your arms and relax.

Repeat exercises 7–10 on your left side – raising your left arm and bending your left leg and leaning on your right side.

TOTAL HEALTH
& FITNESS

BEAUTY

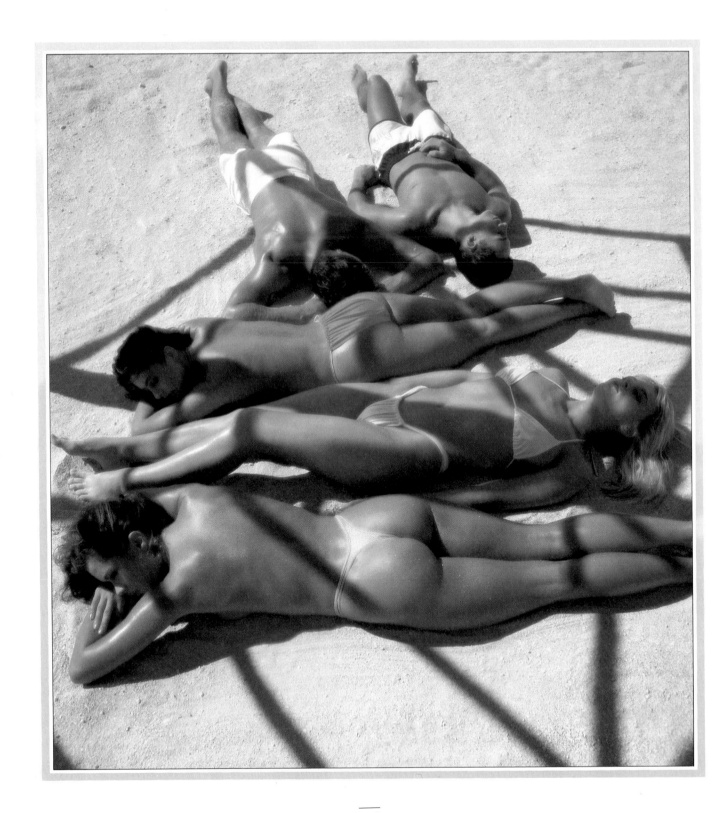

SKIN CARING

Skin is marvellous stuff. There's no magician's mantle that can duplicate its diverse roles of waterproof, overcoat, sunshade, suit of armour and refrigerator; sensitive to the touch of a feather, to temperature and to pain, and able to withstand the wear and tear of three score years and ten, all the while executing its own running repairs!

If you are eating healthily, taking regular exercise and fighting stress with relaxation techniques, you should be well on the way to having

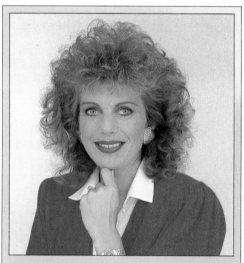

Diet, relaxation and exercise aid healthy skin.

a good-looking skin. But are you really clued up on modern skincare? Here's how to make the most of your complexion, from cleansing and moisturising to facials and problem-solving.

To soap or not to soap? Over the years, the experts seem to have got in all of a lather over what we should do to cleanse our skin properly. Now, the consensus is: *it is OK to wash your face with soap, but use the mildest soap you can find and rinse thoroughly.*

Most skins can take a mild soap and water wash, unless yours is very dry and sensitive. Ordinary alkaline soap is supposed to upset the

pH (the acid/alkaline balance) of the skin, which usually tends towards the acid. However, healthy skin rebounds back to a normal pH of 4.5 in about 10–15 minutes. Although your skin might feel a bit taut after washing, the skin oils rebound in about the same time, too.

But what if it still feels dry and taut after 15 minutes? Switch to a non-soap – a more gentle, rinse-off, creamy cleanser. These are applied like a cream but lather up with water and are then rinsed away, together with make-up, grime and excess oil. They give speedy cleansing, without fuss.

Pay particular attention to rinsing round the hairline, where make-up collects, and around the nose. If you like to use a flannel, be sure to wash it frequently. Highly scented soaps are best kept for the bath and body, not your face, and never use a deodorant soap above your neck.

'Deep cleansing' – strictly a myth?

As the skin is meant to be a barrier, you would not want any cleansing product to penetrate too deeply – nor do they. The word 'deep' – applied to cleansers – is strictly a marketing term. It may actually mean that you're getting a bit too rough on your skin!

What manufacturers mean by 'deep' is 'searching'. Exfoliators or facial scrubs remove surface dead-skin cells – so do face masks. You can exfoliate with grains or with creams with granules, with abrasive sponges, alcohol-containing tonics, even with your face flannel. The beauty products may *claim* to stimulate, but dermatologists say they irritate.

In fact, skin specialists say they see more patients who are suffering the effects of over-doing cleansing rather than because they have not cleansed enough. Burning and stinging is a usual complaint because the skin has been made more sensitive by stripping off the surface protective film.

It is all a matter of degree. When you buff off surface dead-skin cells, your skin often *looks* cleaner and healthier – probably because of blood rushing to the surface. Take the safer route and use exfoliators now and again, not too often, especially if you have a sensitive skin.

Apply exfoliating cleansers to the face with your fingers, rubbing in little circles, avoiding eyes and lips, and paying special attention to more greasy parts such as the forehead, nose, the sides of cheeks nearest the nose, and the chin. Rinse thoroughly.

Cream and lotion cleansers

The traditional way to remove your make-up is with a make-up remover or lotion, followed by skin tonic or freshener on cotton wool. Always considered a soft touch for your face, these products have currently been coming in for more scrutiny. Sometimes they are found wanting, under suspicion of triggering off cosmetic acne and blocked pores. The key word is 'comedogenic'.

Some ingredients in creams and cleansers could indeed trigger, not only sensitive skin reactions, but also spots. Try to buy products that are labelled 'non-comedogenic', or just be vigilant. If you find your skin is breaking out more than usual with your favoured products, perhaps you should change to another brand.

Alcohol is an effective degreasant but can also be an irritant. It is mostly found in the stronger astringents used for greasy skins. Gentle skin tonics and fresheners are alcohol-free. Very dry and sensitive skins cannot use alcohol-based cleansers and may even find water-cleansing too much. These gentle creamy cleansers may be the answer. But remove them carefully with tissues, and use a non-alcoholic gentle freshener on cotton wool as a 'rinse' to wipe away the last traces.

Even if you are careful to wipe away as much of the cleanser as possible, faint traces will still remain, and this can be irritating for the skin. Cleansing lotions and creams are formulated with surfactants, a kind of detergent, and are meant to be taken off – not left on.

Eye make-up removers are useful because they enable you to take off eyeshadow, liner and mascara gently and efficiently. Use a non-oily remover if you wear contact lenses. In any case, take off eye make-up gently with a cotton ball, stroking *up* and out.

And remember, nothing – no skin tonic, astringent, freshener or plain cold water – can close your pores. Would life were that simple! Pores are not doors in the skin that open and close. They are the openings to the hair follicles. Slight irritation can swell the skin and so make the pore openings look less obvious temporarily. Greasy skins often have more coarse and 'open' pores. Dry skins are usually finer with less obvious pores. It is a matter of genetics. You inherit your skin type. But all skin can be improved with consistent care and protection.

A mask of beauty

Giving yourself a home facial now and again makes you feel fresher. Face masks work by means of a mild exfoliating action, stripping off surface dead-skin cells. Clay masks which dry on the skin are grease-absorbing and act better on oily skins. Peel-off masks are more gentle but less cleansing than clay. Moisture masks are non-drying and best for dry and sensitive skins.

Your face will become pinker because of increased blood circulation – when masks dry, they 'pinch' the skin and blood tends to rush to the surface. So it is probably not a good idea to give yourself a facial just before going out.

For oily/combination skins that are tending to look rather muddy, you can try the occasional home facial sauna. Cleanse your face first, then sprinkle some pot-pourri petals and herbs onto about ¾ pint of freshly boiling water in a heat-resistant bowl. Position your head over the bowl and cover your head and the bowl with a towel to allow the steam to penetrate. Keep the attitude about 5–10 minutes. Then cleanse your face again and splash with cool water or just a refreshing toner on cotton wool. Don't do this kind of facial if you have a very sensitive skin or broken veins on your cheeks.

MOISTURISERS – FOR A SOFTER TOUCH

Skin contains about 70 percent water, 10–13 percent of which is within the outer, visible corneal layer. When the water level drops, the result is obvious: our skin tends to look dull, taut and more lined because of dehydration.

Surprisingly, skin dehydration is *not* linked with age or sex. In fact, a man's skin can be just as dry as a woman's. Basic skin water levels are decided at birth. It is environmental factors and chemical interference that make all the difference to keeping the skin soft.

The colder the temperature, the drier your skin becomes, whatever your skin type. When the atmosphere is hot and dry and the humidity low, skin also gets dehydrated. Water diffusing from internal tissues towards the outer layers of skin will not be sufficient to replace that which evaporates from the surface.

As a result you get that taut, dry feeling, and lack of elasticity. 'Chemical interference' is what you actually apply to your skin in the form of cleansers, harsh astringents and face masks. These are factors which could encourage dehydration because they may destroy the natural hydrolipidic film which protects your skin from excessive evaporation of moisture. This film is a natural emulsion which defends your skin against the hostile environment. It also controls gradual water loss, retaining just the right amount of moisture your skin needs.

Moisturisers try to copy Nature's way. They are emulsions with water as a major constituent. Making them is a bit like making mayonnaise: waxy or oily ingredients and water are blended together with emulsifiers to produce a lotion or cream. They work by forming an invisible barrier to prevent water loss. They achieve this, not just by a film of grease alone, but also by aiming to copy the skin's water-holding hydrolipidic film. Modern moisturisers often have added benefits, particularly ultra-violet filters to help prevent sun damage. Many of today's new creams also claim to be 'non-comedogenic' – they will not trigger off spots. 'Non-allergenic' on a moisturiser is self-explanatory.

Most of us need to use a moisturiser each day, although oily/combination skins can get away with the lighter types, applied to neck, cheeks and eye area, and avoiding the very greasiest parts of the face, There are moisturisers . . . and moisturisers. Some last on the skin longer than others. You need to test different products to find one that really suits. New formulae claim anything from 15 to 24 hours' efficacy, so check the small print on the pack!

Choose your type of moisturiser, not only according to your skin type, but also in relation to the climate. Your skin's moisture content varies according to climatic conditions, so when the humidity is high, you will probably need just a light moisturiser. In intense heat or cold, when humidity is low, you'll need a heavy-duty type. Apply moisturiser every morning, before make-up, allowing it to sink into the skin thoroughly. Use moisturiser or skin-conditioning cream at night, particularly if skin is dry or ageing. Some are formulated especially for night use.

SKIN AND AGEING: CAN YOU STOP THE CLOCK?

In the world of beauty, wrinkles are big business. We all get them – and nobody wants them. So any cream or potion which *implies* (the advertising standards authority objects to claims that cannot be proven) that your skin will look more radiant and youthful is on to a good thing.

We have been trying to stop the deteriorating effects of ageing on our skin since the times of the pharaohs. But where once it was poisonous mixtures, including deadly white lead, which claimed the allegiance of the fashion-conscious, today it is the fruits of science, which include collagen, vitamins, 'systems', micro-capsules, thymus extracts and retinoic acid. But can you restore youthfulness from a pot?

That the skin *looks* better after using most creams and lotions, there seems to be no doubt. Sophisticated scientific equipment such as spectro-microscopes, profilometers, ultra-sound and digitised image analysis (borrowed from the US Space Programme, no less) show efficacious results on 'before and after' sections of skin. But is it just cosmetic?

Claims that cells turn over quicker, 'like younger skin', do not make dermatologists enthusiastic. They say that you can make cells reproduce faster if you injure the skin, if you inflame it, slap it, sunburn it or even rub it. Any kind of injury brings forth the repairing response, happily for us. However, many women believe that their skin does look better for using special skin-creams, and who is to say they are wrong? Miracles being thin on the ground these days for most of us, it might be better to look after your skin with reasonably-priced products from well-respected companies who have a reputation to live up to, and good quality control.

Skin deep

As we get older, our metabolism slows down and this affects the skin as much as any other part of the body. The skin is composed basically of three separate layers. The first, the *stratum corneum* – the topmost layer of the epidermis – is made up of bonded, interlocked, horny, dead cells, which form a barrier and are continuously being shed. These compact cells are surrounded by layers of inter-cellular membranes which are made of different lipids. These enable skin to hold water and give cohesion to the dead surface skin cells, providing a flat, luminous effect.

New cells are born in the second or *basal* layer of skin, at the bottom of the epidermis. As they mature, they migrate to the skin surface – the skin renews itself about every 28 days. Don't faint, but most of the dust in your home is made up of flaked-off skin! As we age, these basal epidermal cells reproduce less quickly and efficiently, produce fewer essential components and do not hold water so well.

The deepest layer of skin, the *dermis*, is the thickest, underlying tough and resilient tissue, which cushions the body against injury and provides nutriment to the epidermis, the two top layers. It consists of collagen protein and elastic

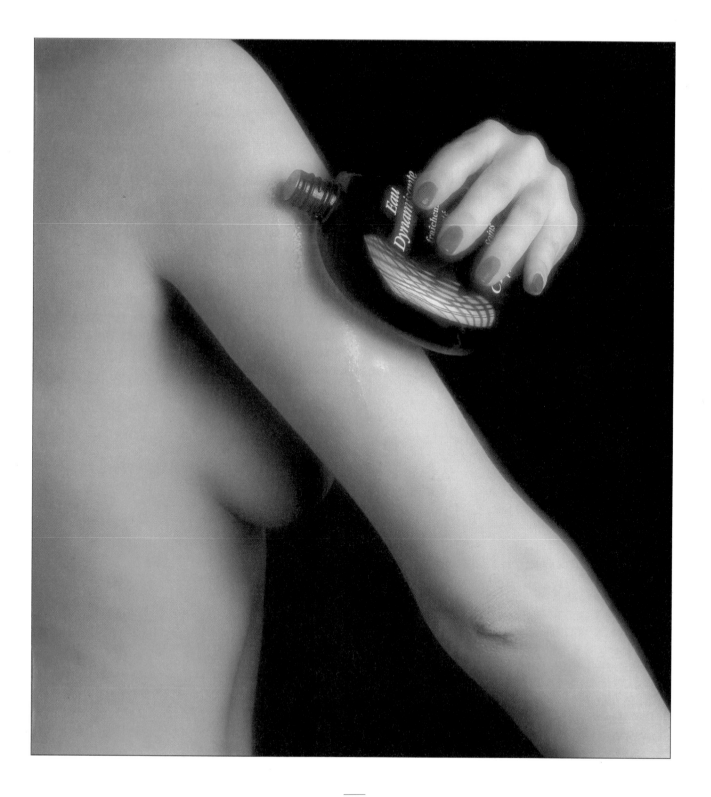

tissue fibres; houses blood, lymphatic and nervous systems; and surrounds the hair follicles and sweat glands. Sunlight penetrates the layers of skin, damaging the collagen and elastic fibres. As a result, the fibroblasts, the cells which produce elastin and collagen, slow down. The upper layers of skin become too big for their filling – and you get wrinkles.

Both sun damage and the natural ageing process contribute to the decline in the capacity of skin to hold moisture effectively: loss of collagen and elastic tissue mean lack of firmness and resilience, while blood vessels in the dermis have more difficulty supplying adequate nutrition to the skin. All this means that, as you get older, your skin becomes thinner. Hello to lines and wrinkles, loss of elasticity, firmness, tone and skin colour.

No wonder we want to find a miracle cream! No-one yet has found a way to halt the ageing process, and until that miracle cream is created and becomes available at the corner shop, the rules for saving your skin are simple:

○ *Stay out of the sun*, or at least use a high-factor suncream (more about suntanning later).
○ *Don't smoke*. Smokers screw up their eyes and lips when they puff a cigarette and this can surely lead to more wrinkles.
○ *Protect your skin from harsh weather*.

WHAT IT MEANS

Reading the label or instruction leaflet which accompanies your skin cream can sometimes seem like trying to understand a foreign language. Here are the key words you may come across and what they mean . . .

Hydrolipidic film A protective natural emulsion on the skin surface made up mostly of natural oil and water.

Hypertrophy Increase in size when referring to skin cells.
Cutaneous degradation Breakdown of skin tissue.
Non-comedogenic Doesn't encourage spots and blackheads.
Desquamation A process in which the outer layer of the skin is removed by buffing, rubbing or sloughing, descaling or exfoliation.
Microtopography A microscopical study of selected parts of the body and their relation to surrounding structures.
Stereoprofilometry A skin imprint technique which manufacturers use to try and prove their creams give good results. An adhesive resin is applied to the skin surface. This is peeled off and examined under a microscope. A fine needle is passed over the mould to get a surface profile of the skin so it is possible to prove if wrinkles are less deep than before.

PROBLEM SKIN

Although we tend to get most spots in our teens, we are liable to get the odd pimple even after 40, and 'cosmetic acne' can cause distress at any age.

Acne may be a case of a few spots and blackheads, or it can be a highly distressing skin disease with redness, inflammation, pimples and even scarring. It is all a matter of degree. Acne in adolescents often appears around the age of 12 or 13 in girls and about 16 in boys, and it peaks at 17–18 in girls and 19 in boys, who suffer more acutely. It is linked to hormones, the male androgen hormones being responsible for spot and grease problems in both sexes. The changing balance of these male hormones over-activate the oil glands, most notably on the face but also on the upper back.

ON THE SPOT

Doctors have been puzzling over the cause of acne for many years and trying to find a cure. However there is still no sure preventive treatment, although much progress has been made in acne therapy. If you have a bad case of spots, do see your doctor. You can forget old wives' tales about it clearing up 'when you get married' or 'growing out of it'. Acne spots may well lessen as you get older and your hormones settle down, but by that time, you may have some scarring.

Pimples can cause much anguish, so it pays to learn as much as you can about your skin, and to get the help of your doctor or a dermatologist at a hospital skin clinic.

The first signs of a problem start with greasy skin and a few blackheads or whiteheads on nose, cheeks and forehead, indicating the rise to maturity of previously insignificant grease glands. Your shiny skin is caused by oil which surfaces via the hair follicles or shafts (otherwise known as the skin's pores), into which the sebaceous glands secrete sebum.

One acne theory has it that an enzyme deficiency permits testosterone (the male sex hormone present in both men and women) to run riot, allowing it to be converted within the skin into a by-product called *dihydrotestosterone* (DHT) which over-stimulates the sebaceous glands. If you have high levels of DHT, you are more likely to suffer acne, get excessive facial hair, have more developed breasts and sometimes lack of periods, than women whose hormone levels are balanced.

There could be a genetic link – an inherited sensitivity. Hair follicles or pore ducts are the battleground for the Spot War. Besides the over-abundance of grease, pores can also become blocked by dead skin cells through an acceleration in cell production. This can dam up a pore until eventually there is leakage into surrounding skin tissue, producing the familiar red bumps, pimples, and in the worst acne cases, cysts and infected abscesses.

Blackheads are pores blocked by dirty grease or dead skin, but whiteheads are worse. They are closed and there is no opening you can unblock easily. The blockage leads to inflammation and pussy infection. Normal skin bacteria breaks down into irritating free-fatty acids.

You can get acne spots for other than hormonal reasons, too. Excessive humidity is a trigger – especially if you use any rich face creams or cosmetics that contain comedogenic ingredients. Contact with oil or oily machinery can lead to pimples, while certain drugs used for the treatment of disease may cause acne as a side effect. Steroids, which are so helpful in other ways, can produce extensive acne on face, chest and back.

You may get spots because of pre-menstrual hormone fluctuation or through taking the Pill – especially the low-oestrogen, high progesterone or progesterone-only varieties. Even emotional stress can be a trigger to finely-tuned glands responsible for the maintenance of hormone levels.

NATURE VS NURTURE

Sunbathing is traditionally supposed to help spotty skins because the sun's drying tendency unblocks greasy pores and encourages quicker cell renewal. But although spots may seem to improve at the beginning, post-holiday, you may well find you are getting eruptions. This is because the skin responds to sunlight by thickening as a protection, and this leads to blocked follicles, beginning the spot-cycle all over again.

Instead of conventional peeling medications such as resorcinol or benzoylperoxide, some dermatologists are now prescribing a more powerful peeling medication based on retinoic acid, a synthetic derivative of vitamin A. This ingredient has been discovered to also have the effect of making skin look younger; extensive testing is being carried out. Antibiotics are also prescribed for acne treatment and need to be given for several months at a time to be effective. Tetracycline and erythromycin have been used for years, though minocycline is now increasingly considered as a preferable and safe alternative.

Acne responds slowly and drugs need time to work. They help to cut down the number of acne bacteria in the blocked-up grease glands and reduce painful inflammation. Side effects may include vaginal thrush, sensitivity to sunlight and even depression or bowel problems. Dosage and timing need to be carefully monitored. Doctors sometimes consider adjusting the hormone balance in girls with long-term persistent acne, using a chemical which blocks the action of male hormones in the body, combined with the female hormone oestrogen.

Over-the-counter medicated skin cleansers and washes can help to control superficial grease but as the problem acne bacteria are inside the follicle, they cannot get rid of spots on their own.

It's not dirt that causes acne. Dirty faces are no more prone to spots than clean faces, say dermatologists. So 'deep cleansing' is not really relevant. Soap and water washing helps to remove surface grease temporarily. Any so-called 'dirt' you may see on a piece of cotton wool after rubbing your skin with astringent or lotion may just be the remnants of make-up or skin cells, which are flaking off all the time.

For some skin conditions, such as eczema-related spots, doctors may prescribe a tar shampoo, and this can be very effective, both for scalp flakiness and for your skin.

It is worth reiterating to look out for cosmetic ranges labelled 'non-comedogenic'. They will be less likely to trigger off more spots. Above all, treat your skin gently. Don't attack your skin with strong, abrasive exfoliators and 'clarifiers'. Some cleansers help loosen simple blackheads, but are unsuitable for whiteheads, inflamed pimples or cysts.

A spot is not . . .
. . . *a punishment* for eating chocolate and rich foods. They might not be doing your figure or teeth a lot of good, but there is no proof that they trigger acne. However, if you have noticed that your spots seem more extravagant following a choc-binge, then perhaps you will have to test and see for yourself whether it makes any difference. We are all individual.

. . . *just a teen problem*. About 50% of teenagers do develop acne and about 5% of women continue to suffer spot problems into late 20's and early 30's. But you can be more spot-prone pre-menstruation because of hormone levels fluctuating, and you can have spot problems after pregnancy and the menopause. One survey discovered that 31% of spot sufferers had blemishes for 3–5 years, and 14% for more than 10 years.

. . . *caused by dirt*. It is not bad hygiene or insufficient cleansing that causes or encourages your spots. But fierce scrubbing and harsh degreasing can certainly traumatise your skin, say experts, and lead to more problems.

ACNE ROSACEA

This is a spotty problem that is different from teenage acne. There are no blackheads and the symptoms include a flush, mainly on cheeks, nose and forehead with perhaps some swelling of the nose. It is most usually seen in women aged 30–50, and gets worse in hot, humid weather, in the cold, and following hot drinks, eating highly seasoned foods or a period of emotional stress.

A course of low-dose tetracycline antibiotic therapy is often effective, but topical steroid creams should be avoided. Never borrow a friend's spot treatment.

SPOT RELIEF

How to help yourself

○ See your doctor if spots are severe and he may send you to a dermatologist. If you get the odd spot, then self-medication and care should be enough.

○ Never pick or squeeze spots. You can get cross infection or push inflammation deeper into the tissues, resulting in scarring.

○ Try a peeling or drying medication. Some contain sulphur or resorcinol; others, the powerful benzoyl peroxide. They help to unblock pores, breaking down the plug of oil and debris, penetrating into the pore to kill bacteria and reduce inflammation, and encourage flaking off of dead skin cells. However, some chemical peelers may also be an irritant and have the unfortunate effect of giving you irritated red patches as a side effect. But this redness and flaking is temporary. You may need to reduce the amount you use. Read instructions carefully.

SUN AND SNOW

The fact that sunlight is damaging to our skin is now universally agreed. But that does not stop us yearning for a glamorous tan. To gain the desired bronze, we often endure burnt shoulders and peeling noses, only to find that the colour fades all too quickly, often a couple of weeks after the holiday.

Ideally, the best thing we can do for our complexions is to stay out of the sun altogether. On the other hand, it seems such a shame not to enjoy the outdoor life in summer. You can get brown without burning, and restrict sun damage, if you just take a bit of care and be scrupulous about protection.

Be realistic about your skin type. If you have a fair, sensitive skin, your genetic capability of tanning may be limited and you are most at risk from burning and all the nasty effects of too much sunlight, including skin cancer. But even Med-type, non-sensitive skins need sun-protection against premature ageing.

THE GOLDEN RULES

○ Limit your sunbathing on the first day of the holiday. Don't just rush onto the beach and stretch out for hours and hours. The sunburn redness may not reveal itself until later in the day and by that time, the damage will be done and could ruin thё rest of your stay. Whatever your skin type, do use a high-factor sunscreen and reapply it frequently.

○ Avoid the hottest time of the day, when the sun's rays are directly overhead and at their most powerful and harmful. That means from about 12.00 until 2.30pm. These are the hours when burning ultra-violet B rays are strongest. It's safer to sunbathe earlier in the morning or later in the afternoon, when there is less UVB about but enough ultra-violet A rays to help you get brown.

○ Never fall asleep in direct sunlight. Remember that even if the place you choose to snooze is well-shaded, the shadows may shift before you awake. Follow the locals, when abroad, and have a siesta indoors.

○ Be aware of reflection. Your skin is being bombarded with sunrays which are scattered and reflected off other surfaces. In water, at least 40% of UV radiation is transmitted to a depth of about 20 inches, which means that it is easy to get burned when swimming.

Snow reflects most light, 86%; sand reflects 17%, water 5% and even grass 3%. Altitude, too, makes a big difference to how quickly you can burn. With each 300-metre increase in height, the burning potential of sunlight increases about 4%. So the higher you are, the more exposure to damaging rays, which is why skiing is such a high-risk for sunburns.

○ Don't forget the bits and pieces – shoulders, lips, noses, neck, feet, backs of knees. Your lips have no natural moisturising ability so need frequent application of protective balm or stick. Your feet can get burned when patches of skin are exposed when you wear sandals.

THE BEST TAN PLAN

Use a sunscreen all day every day, and go for the higher factor numbers. The best and longest-lasting tans are acquired slowly – quick tans are usually fast burns and peel off in a trice.

Apply a sunscreen before you go out into the sunlight. Take time to massage it thoroughly into your skin. Use a water-resistant variety if you

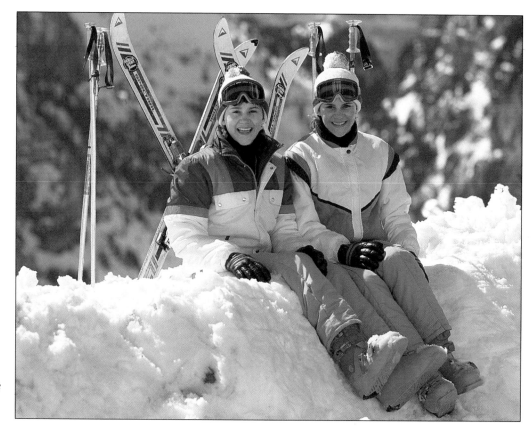

A tan is healthy only as long as you give your skin adequate protection from damaging rays and in the mountains the sun can be particularly strong.

are in-and-out of the sea and pool. But whatever you choose, reapply it frequently throughout the day. Water, towels, sweat and sand all tend to rub it off.

Assess your skin type and be advised by the following good counsel:

Sun sensitive

You often have a fair skin and light-coloured eyes, though your hair colour may vary. Red-heads are particularly vulnerable, but so are those of Celtic origin with dark hair, very pale skins and pale blue or light grey eyes. Yours is the skin most at risk from sunburn, premature ageing and skin cancer, and you need the strongest protection. Skimping on the sunfilter

will not help you to brown any quicker but can leave you sore and damaged.

But remember, you can only go brown if your skin has the ability to do so. Not everyone can. In which case, you can use a fake tan, or be pale and pretty, and thankful that your skin is going to stay less wrinkled for longer!

Choose a sun protection factor of 15 or more for the first few days. Eventually you can use a factor 8 or 10, but be guided by the location and the sun intensity. Wear a hat and keep a shirt handy. Build up your time in the sun gradually – start with half an hour or so. Even with a sunfilter, avoid midday sun because the intense heat can quickly leave your skin hot, tight and dehydrated.

Less sensitive

You probably have dark blonde, mid-brown or darker hair and mid-toned eyes, not too light or too dark. Your skin tans eventually but can burn on the way, if you are not careful.

Choose a factor 8–10 for about the first five days, but be guided by sun intensity and location. Even the less sensitive need a high factor in very intense sunlight, or if you are at very high altitude. Once you have some tan, you can switch to a factor 5–6, but save lower factors (nothing lower than 3 or 4) until the last few days of a 2-week holiday, if you have a tan.

If you love sports and the sun is very hot, wear a white T-shirt, when windsurfing or water-skiing both to reflect the glare and to keep you cooler.

Natural brownies

You probably have a darker or olive skin and a natural in-built tanning ability. The darker your skin, the more protected it is, but most skins still need to use a sunfilter, especially during the first five days. Even for you the sun can cause premature ageing, although you might not see the damage until years later.

Choose a factor 5–6 at least to start, and switch to 3–4 later. Leave the factor 2 tanning oil until the last few days.

GOING FOR THE BURN

When your skin is burned, your body responds in the same way as it does to any other injury: going into 'over-drive' to quickly replace the burnt areas with new skin. Then the damaged skin peels off.

A slight burn can cause a pale pink colour which may appear between 6–24 hours after exposure and can take 1–3 days to disappear, but may not cause peeling. If your skin is bright pink and slightly painful, you have got a definite burn. This may appear between 2–12 hours after exposure and last 3 days, with light peeling.

A nastier burn leaves you very red, with some pain and swelling several hours after exposure. It can take 3 days to disappear and is followed by complete peeling.

The worst kind of burn gives painful blisters and general skin damage within about an hour after exposure. This can require a week to die down, and is followed by severe peeling that leaves no brown pigment remaining.

Soothing remedies: take aspirin – it inhibits prostaglandin formation (sunburn releases it in the body) and will considerably reduce soreness and redness if taken early enough. Keep an after-sun soothing preparation handy. Cooling gels with aloe vera can do much to relieve discomfort.

Folk recipes to try: take a lukewarm bath with two cups of cider vinegar or some bicarbonate of soda added. Or add a cup each of vinegar and cooking oil. Soak for 15 minutes, then pat yourself dry gently. Mix equal parts of baking powder and water and pat on the sunburnt areas. Leave for half an hour before rinsing with tepid water. Spread on slices of cooling cucumber or cold bags.

NOT SO RASH

Heat rashes, prickly heat and allergic reactions affect many sunbathers – in fact, about a third of the population seems to suffer. There are at least 20 types of sun allergy, caused by UVA and possibly UVB radiation being absorbed by a chemical in the skin. This triggers chemical changes in your body, which reacts as if threatened by a foreign substance. Your body tries to get rid of the 'stranger' by calling up the immune system, causing a *photoallergic* reaction.

The sun can also act as the catalyst to many everyday substances which are stored in the skin and can be stimulated into an allergic response by deep-penetrating UVA rays. Low-calorie drinks (it's the sweetener that does it), citrus fruit, antibiotics and fragrances can lead to problems. Some people are even unlucky enough to get a reaction from their suntan protective preparation.

Sun rashes can appear hours after exposure but may take days or even weeks to disappear. If you find you normally get a rash every time you go in the sun, do see your doctor earlier in the year. He may be able to prescribe some therapy that can help.

Avoid the sun in the middle of the day, use high-factor sunscreens (always with UVA filter as well as UVB), drink mineral water rather than sweetened soft drinks, and avoid deodorant or perfumed soaps, cosmetics or toiletries prior to sunbathing.

FAKE TANS

Tan cosmetics and delayed-action tanners give you a bronze glow without the health risks. Delayed-action bronzers based on dehydroxy-acetone are well proven and safe, combining with the skin's amino acids to produce a tan colour after 3–5 hours. You cannot guarantee what the resulting shade will be, though – you build up depth with subsequent layers – and you can get tell-tale streaking if you are not very careful with application.

Large pores may collect colouring pigment and look darker, while the horny, dry skin on elbows, knees and backs of heels may also grab the colour. Prepare your skin beforehand by moisturising all over, every day, for at least a week before you use the fake tan.

PROLONGING YOUR TAN

Untanned skin takes time for the natural melanin pigment to be triggered off by sunrays and to rise to the surface to make you look brown. Melanin pigmentation reaches its maximum about the 20th day of sun exposure. But you seem to lose the tan very quickly once you are back at work.

How to keep up the colour? Use a fake tan – a tan foundation or tinted moisturiser will make your face look more glowing for quite a while after your holiday. Don't scrub too much in the bath or shower, and switch to a more-moisturising shower gel or 'skin shampoo' instead of drying soap. Choose bath oils rather than bubble-baths. Apply plenty of cream or body lotion every night.

What about sunbeds? As UVA rays penetrate deepest into the skin and are linked to both skin ageing and irritable skin eruptions, artificial UVA solariums are not recommended by dermatologists. If you must, don't have any more than 20 sessions a year, say the experts. For your skin's sake, it would be better not to have any.

I heard of one 35-year-old secretary who bought a special offer at a solarium, soaked up 50 half-hour sessions of artificial sun in ten weeks, and found her shins covered with large, dark, irregular freckles that remained and spread.

Sunbed-users get reddening, itching and dryness, and 10% develop photosensitisation and polymorphic light eruptions (like prickly heat). New research has shown that UVA causes severe ageing changes in the skin of mice and it is virtually certain that humans get degenerative changes, too, and perhaps acceleration of skin cancers.

PATCHY PIGMENTATION

Giant freckles, called chloasma, sometimes appear on the face or neck in sunlight if you are pregnant or taking the combined Pill. It is thought to be a reaction to the sex hormones oestrogen and progesterone.

Another form of patchy skin pigmentation occurs – usually on the face and neck – as a response to the aromatic oils in perfumes. Never spray or dab on perfume before going in sunlight.

Chloasma nearly always goes away of its own accord when the high levels of circulating hormones return to normal. But do see your doctor. You may need a change of Pill. Some sufferers find a sunblock cream may help.

THE DANGERS

We now know that too much sun ages the skin, destroys elastic tissue and collagen, causes patchy pigmentation, rashes and wrinkles. But these are cosmetic effects. Much worse is the link between serious sunburn and deadly skin cancer.

Cases of malignant melanoma have more than doubled in the last 10 years in countries with a fair-skinned population. As more of us get opportunities to take one or more holidays abroad in the sun each year, the chances of getting a melanoma are increasing, say doctors.

Dermatologists recommend: stay inside when the sun rays are strongest and make sure you wear a factor 15 or more on exposed skin. Since sunscreens offer relative, not absolute protection, most of us can get a tan using high-protection filters. It is thought that sudden exposure to intense sunlight is a trigger to melanoma, and young office workers are typical victims. You are most at risk if you strip off to bask in blazing sun after a year covered up.

Melanomas can appear anywhere on the body, but the legs are most often affected. It takes the form of a dark, slightly raised lump – perhaps an existing mole which enlarges and bleeds. If you notice any mole changing in character, a new mole appearing, or large dark freckles showing up on your skin, do see your doctor. About 70% of cases start on normal skin which has had sun damage, and 30% develop from moles which are present at birth.

The majority of other types of skin cancer are the result of continued exposure to sunlight over a long period of time. Unlike melanomas, they are slow growing and non-invasive and are readily curable if treated early.

COLD COMFORT

In winter, skin has other problems to contend with – dry cold is extremely dehydrating and skin can become very dry indeed with central heating and lack of humidity.

Pay particular attention to moisturising. Each morning apply a layer of moisturiser, allow it to sink in, then put on a second layer. Don't forget your neck, lips and eyes. A make-up base is not only a flattering cosmetic, it is also a protection against the cold and wind. Use a moisturised foundation if your skin is normal-to-dry.

If you are prone to thread veins on the cheeks, extremes of temperature are not good – wrap a scarf round your face when you go out in chill temperatures and cold winds, and don't sit too near the fire when you come in. Use a heavy-duty moisturiser and a good covering base. A green (yes green) tinged under-base or moisturiser helps to tone down a ruddy complexion.

the BODY BEAUTIFUL

The skin on your face and body may seem the same but facial skin actually has more sebaceous glands to secrete natural oil and keep skin supple. It also has a looser cell structure, which makes penetration by moisturisers into the top layer easier. Body skin has fewer oil-producing glands, leaving large areas of skin without natural lubrication. It has a more compact cellular structure so it is difficult for moisturisers to work well on the epidermis.

If you neglect to moisturise your body skin, particularly on the lower legs, you get a sort of crazy-paving cracked look over the shins, and the skin on your elbows and heels can become callused and thickened. So don't let skincare end at the neck. Your body skin needs care and attention, too, and will repay pampering by looking and feeling softer and smoother.

A LOOK AT BATHTIME

Having a long soak in the tub is enjoyable and therapeutic: your muscles relax, your mind feels

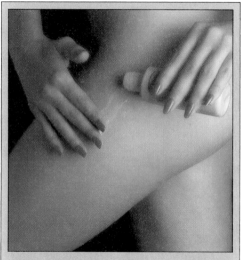

Sweet smells and oils lubricate the outer skin

more tranquillised as you let go after the stresses of the day. Immersion in water is less beneficial for the skin than for the woman, however.

A long bath can dehydrate, leaving your skin feeling taut and looking wrinkled. Especially in hard water areas, the longer the bath and the hotter its temperature, the greater the dehydration is likely to be. Showers are more invigorating than calming and can have a stimulating effect on your skin . . . and your mood.

Also the stronger the solution of minerals and salts in your bathwater, the more moisture your skin loses, however delightful it might make you feel to bathe in bubbles. So don't use detergent-based bubble-bath every day, and go more for bath oils than salts.

Soaps are also efficient 'defatting' agents which encourage dryness. So come clean with mild soaps or non-soap moisturising 'body shampoos' and bath or shower gels.

After your bath lavish on lots of body conditioner or moisturising lotion, massaging it into your skin from the tips of your toes to your shoulders, up to your neck.

Rougher stuff: If your body skin looks goose-pimply and sluggish, sloughing off dead surface skin cells with an abrasive mitt or exfoliating product can make a big difference to texture and touch.

Body scrubs contain 'polishing' grains, which you massage in lightly with circular movements, before rinsing. Apply once or twice a week, especially to backs of arms and thighs, your feet, elbows and knees.

Friction gloves, or friction sponges and back-straps, loofahs and back brushes, give more abrasive treatment. Give your skin the occasional stimulating body brush-up, concentrating especially on the more oily and potentially spotty areas like your back, between the shoulders.

Only tougher skins can take the famous spa seasalt scrub: you rub granular salt onto the rough areas of skin with circular movements, rinse off, then apply body lotion.

GIVING A MASSAGE

Having a salon massage is one of life's little treats. But it is possible to give yourself a massage at home, after your bath, using a rich lubricating cream or body oil. Or for a treat, try an aromatherapy oil.

There are three main groups of techniques: *effleurage*, which consists of skin 'rolling', picking up and kneading; and *stroking*, which includes vibrations. Another series of movements is grouped under the heading *tapotement*. These are the pounding, clapping and slapping.

Give yourself a massage either standing up or sitting down on a towel. Tie your hair back out of the way. All strokes should be made in the direction of the heart, pushing blood towards it. You can use one or both hands.

Use hand-over-hand stroking movements on legs from ankle to thigh. Alternately press and release pressure with palms, gradually wriggling the hands fairly vigorously along the muscles.

Do kneading movements on the body, placing the hands palms down on the back with the fingers meeting at waist level, thumbs pointing forwards. Knead comfortably up and down from side to side, then knead the sides of the waist.

For skin rolling, seize the flesh between thumb and forefinger and lift it away from the bone. Drop and repeat, moving your hand along, grasping handfuls of flesh. Do not dig in.

Stroking is sensuous. It can be more soothing.

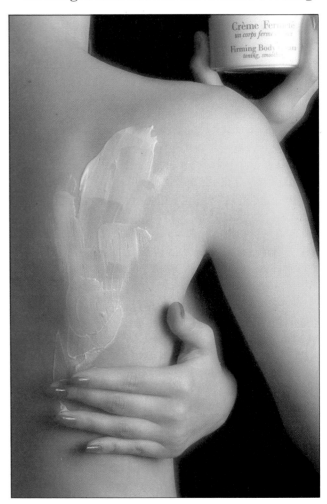

A herbal cream or fragrant oil gives a soothing massage

Step by step

○ Legs and feet: Hold a foot in one hand and gently pull the toes with the other hand. Using your thumbs, massage the instep from the toes upwards. Swivel the foot slowly in a circular movement to the right, then to the left.

Bend one leg and effleurage the calf, gently but firmly stroking. Then use the palm of the hand to knead the main muscle, using a slight 'wringing' movement on the inside and outside of the calf.

'Pick' the inside and outside of the leg apart, using fingers and thumb (don't pinch). Use effleurage strokes on thigh, followed by kneading and wringing. Repeat with other foot and leg.

○ Stomach and ribs: Be careful around the tummy area. Massage by pressing gently with palms of hands, then knead with fingertips gently around the navel. 'Pick' flesh around the waist and effleurage the ribs.

○ Arms: Massage gently but firmly, pushing the skin up the arm away from you. Do effleurage, followed by 'plucking' and kneading movements. Effleurage the shoulders and press gently.

○ The back: Naturally, you cannot do your own as soothingly as someone else doing it for you. But reach as far as you can. Stroke and knead the back of the shoulders where muscles tend to get knotted. Try to do firm rhythmic movements. With your thumbs, gently knead the small of your back. Alternate kneading with effleurage strokes.

FIGHTING THE FUZZ

Too much hair in the wrong place can be an embarrassment and a nuisance. But just what is considered too hairy in one society may be perfectly OK in another. It is social custom as well as genetics.

Removing body hair has been a custom for centuries. When Ovid wrote his text book on the art of loving nearly 2,000 years ago, he advised women that 'no rude goat should find his way beneath your arms, and that your legs be not rough with bristling hairs.'

Hairiness under arms and in the pubic region is normal, of course. But just how much hair grows there is individual. A few coarse hairs may grow round the nipples or between the breasts. Some very feminine women have hair growing in the small of their backs, while a faint moustache or dark downy hair down the sides of the face are not uncommon.

Latin looks and darker, more obvious body hair go together. Blondes and redheads are luckier in this respect. So what can you do about getting rid of it?

Reach for the bleach

A mild degree of hairiness on arms, legs or upper lip, when the hair is very fine, not coarse, can be disguised by lightening with a cream bleach. Be sure to buy one specially designed for the body and face – don't use a hair bleach.

A close shave

For quickness, there's nothing to beat shaving your legs and under arms, but as you slice off the hair at skin level, you soon get prickly regrowth. Shaving does not, of course, cause hair to grow any thicker or quicker or there would not be any bald men about!

The secret of successful shaving is to soften the skin with water and soap, or a shaving preparation. Spread on lather evenly and shave first with downward strokes, then relather and shave in the opposite direction. Shave legs with long smooth strokes from ankle to knee and from knee to thigh. Rinse and pat dry. Electric shavers are fast, convenient and safe, although some users find dry shaving takes some getting used to. But after any kind of shave, use a moisturising lotion on your skin.

Cream depilatories

These are creams, lotions, sprays and mousses which dissolve away unwanted hair just below skin level, using chemicals such as calcium thioglycollate. This dissolves hair by breaking the sulphur bonds of the keratin, the protein from which hair is made.

The process is fast – about 4–6 minutes for the cream and 6–8 minutes for the mousse – and as it dissolves hair a little below the surface of the skin, the result is often smoother, without stubble, and a slower regrowth then shaving.

The only problem is that it is messy and somewhat smelly, though much less so than it used to be. Test for skin sensitivity first. Never apply a depilatory cream to inflamed or broken skin, or shortly before or after using soap, deodorant or a perfumed product. Irritation or, at worst, infection can result.

The big strip

Waxing, which is wholesale plucking essentially, removes hair from the roots and the results last longer – often for weeks. After years of regular waxing, the hair follicles may give up the unequal struggle and not grow back. But this can just mean patchy regrowth, with bald patches, not the whole leg of hair disappearing. And, as the hairs on head and body are all at different stages of the hair growth cycle, waxing does not always mean that some hair doesn't grow back quickly – it may have been just under the skin just waiting to pop out!

In beauty salons, you can have hair waxed with traditional hot wax, which is applied with a spatula in sections and pulled off in strips quickly, taking the hairs with it. Or you can have 'warm' or 'cool' wax. With this method, a thin layer of tepid wax is spread on the skin. Cotton strips are pressed on top, then ripped off. Cool waxing is said to be quickest, but advocates of hot wax say that it is much more efficient.

At home, you can used pre-waxed strips. Not all hairs come off in one go however, and you may need to go over sections again and again. For best results, some products are recommended to be used after dusting your skin with talc first. Don't use strips within two hours of bathing, as hot water makes skin more sensitive.
○ Tips for success: apply strips of wax to the hair, then strip off in the opposite direction of hair growth. Don't pull strips straight up or you may irritate skin and break off hair. Use one quick ripping motion parallel to the skin and close to it, holding skin taut.

Does it hurt? That depends on your pain threshold. It is something like ripping off a plaster. If you do it quickly, there's nothing to it.

Skin electrolysis

This is the only permanent method of hair removal, and even electrolysis does not necessarily work in one go. Treatments may need to be repeated over months. As it is an expensive and time-consuming treatment, it is best kept for smaller areas, such as the upper lip.

A quick rip off

Tweezers are invaluable for removing odd hairs. A quick pull, and it is out from the roots. Use fine-chisel edged tweezers rather than points which can damage the skin. Keep antiseptic cream handy just in case.

Body hair growing untidily or in odd places can be removed by waxing in a salon, if you can't reach it. If you feel embarrassed, get to know the beautician first, by trying a leg or arm wax. Rest assured, they have seen far hairier clients than you!

Try having underarm hair waxed, too, as well as your legs. It isn't so painful and hair removed from the roots in this area becomes very discouraged. Hair may well grow back finer and more sparse.

WATCH YOUR STEP

Are you ashamed of your feet or can you bare them with pride? Almost all of us start life with trouble-free feet, but by the time we reach 20, there are inevitably some problems.

The main problem is shoes. Too short, too tight, too pointed or whatever, they take their toll on your feet. Friction and pressure from shoes are responsible for two of the most common foot ailments: corns and calluses. The skin is sandwiched between the bone and the shoe and continuous irritation and chaffing causes skin to build up a protective bulwark until it is a thickened layer of dead, horny tissue.

With corns, the build-up is cone-shaped, with the pointed end – the nucleus – facing downwards. When it presses on a nerve, it causes pain. There are two types of corn, the hard variety – which usually develops on the tips or top of the toes – and the soft corn that builds up between the toes.

Calluses grow on the ball of the foot and do not have a nucleus. But the thick, hardened layers of dead skin sometimes press on the nerve, causing a burning sensation when you walk.

To prevent problems you must take care in buying shoes that fit well. It is asking for trouble to wear shoes with heels over 2½ inches high for long periods. Too short tights or stockings can also harm feet.

Treat calluses by rubbing with a callus file, a pumice stone, or a hard-skin remover. Corns are better dealt with by a chiropodist. Over-the-counter remedies sometimes lead to skin sensitivity. Stubborn patches of dry skin can be removed with a rough skin remover cream, rubbed in, then rinsed off. Massage cream into feet to prevent hard skin and to make your feet softer and smoother. There are now special preparations, based on herbs such as peppermint and rosemary, just for feet.

Foot revivers

Tone your foot muscles. Stand with the feet together and slowly raise up on tiptoes, then lower the heels down again. Or try to pick up marbles with your toes. Walk barefoot – when it is safe to do so. Wriggle your toes, then alternately curl them up tight for a count of five and stretch them out to another five count.

Stand barefoot on the edge of a step. Hold onto the bannister rail and lower your heels down slowly, then slowly rise on tiptoe. Repeat four times. Sit on a chair, slip off your shoes, and keeping your legs as still as possible, slowly revolve each foot in turn, drawing an imaginary circle with your toes.

A regular pedicure

Do your nails after your bath, when nails are softer. Clip toenails straight across – never cut too far down at the sides as this leads to ingrowing toenails. Smooth over the edges with an emery board.

Dip a cotton bud into cuticle-remover and go round each cuticle, then push back with a rubber-tipped hoofstick. Don't cut cuticles. Rinse off the remover afterwards.

Remove hard skin with a file or hard-skin stone, then use a foot cream. Apply a cuticle cream to each nail and rub it in to soften. Clean under each nail.

If you are going to apply nail polish, first swab each nail free of grease with a little remover on cotton wool. Apply a base coat, then two coats of varnish, allowing each coat to dry thoroughly before applying the next one. Keep your toes apart with cotton wool, tissues or rubber toe-spacers. When varnish is completely dry, apply a final top coat of colourless varnish.

Don't keep painting over chipped or worn polish. Clean off the old polish thoroughly and then apply the new. Let your nails 'breathe' *without* polish occasionally.

HELPING HANDS

Your hands and nails are a reflection of your well-being, revealing your age, the kind of work you do, even your self-esteem or nervousness.

Like your hair, nails are primarily composed of keratin, a fibrous, porous protein, whose cells stretch when nails are exposed to water. Constant wetting makes nails soft and opaque, and chemical detergents and varnish removers decrease levels of moisture in the nail. All this leads to swelling and shrinkage of keratin cells, and the bonds that hold together the nail weaken, causing brittleness.

Though nails are lifeless, the nail matrix – the 'womb' of the nail, from which it grows – is richly supplied with blood capillaries and nerve endings. The half moon or *lunala* separates the living nail, which is below the cuticle, from the nail you can see.

Each fingernail grows about an half inch every three months, and toenails about a third of that rate. Growth varies with individuals, however, and is said to vary between winter and summer.

Are you a nail biter?

It takes a tremendous effort to stop, so:
○ Be determined. Try bribing yourself.
○ Keep an emery board handy in case of nail snags, so your teeth do not get to them first!
○ Start by allowing one nail to grow and take pride in it. Then grow a second.
○ Apply a bitter-tasting nail-biting deterrent.

How to handle a manicure

A regular home manicure need not take too long, but it can make all the difference to the condition and looks of hands and nails.
1 Remove old polish with varnish-remover and cotton wool. Apply the pad, soaked in remover, to the nail for a second or two; allow to soften before swabbing off the polish thoroughly.

2 Use a fine emery board to shape the nails into rounded ovals, filing from side to centre in one direction only. See-sawing leads to rough edges. Do not file nails too far down at the sides.
3 To soak or not to soak? Although manicurists in salons often do, the new thinking is don't; soap and water may soften the cuticles but can be a cause of brittle nails. Apply cuticle remover all round the nail and gently push down the cuticles with a rubber-tipped hoof stick, a cotton bud, or cotton wool wrapped round an orange stick.
4 Clean under the nails, too. Wash off cuticle remover.
5 Apply cuticle cream and massage round the nails thoroughly.
6 Swab the nails with nail-varnish remover to take away any grease.
7 Apply a base coat to fill in ridges and give a smoother surface.
8 Apply nail varnish, at least two coats.
9 Seal with a top coat of colourless varnish for a longer-lasting shine.

Hand savers

Too much varnish remover can make nails brittle. So top up when you can, rather than stripping off old varnish and starting again.

Kitchen chemicals, such as detergents, are bad for nails because they strip away natural oils. Apply a barrier cream for dirty, wet jobs, or use rubber gloves.

Always keep hand cream available in kitchen and bathroom and rub it in frequently.

HAIR LINES

Hair is the ultimate fashion accessory, a means to express our individuality, a flattering frame to the face – and foliage behind which we sometimes hide! Though it is dead the minute it leaves the scalp, your hair has a lot to put up with. It soon shows ill treatment, as well as responding to conditioning and care.

Hair is a marvellous natural fibre – you could almost compare it to pure silk thread. But it is, in fact, a form of protein called keratin, similar in composition to our finger and toenails. The basic material of hair comes from amino acids, and to ensure that cell production continues, the blood supply at the bottom of the hair follicle transports the amino acids, hormones and nutrients required for hair growth. So a poor diet can eventually have an effect on your hair condition.

There are about 100,000 hairs on the scalp – blondes have least, brunettes most – and hair grows about half an inch a month. Each hair goes through distinct stages of growth. There is a period of growing, and a period of resting before

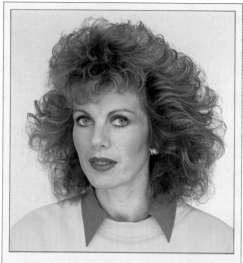

Tender loving care makes all the difference

the hair falls out and a new hair grows in its place. How long you can grow your hair varies – it is probably influenced by genetics. But there is nothing you can do to make it grow longer than it is programmed to do by your body chemistry.

Each hair is made up of three layers: the cuticle on the outside is made up of protective overlapping scales. When these scales lie close to the hair shaft, they provide a light-reflecting surface that makes hair look glossy. When the scales are lifted or broken because of damage, hair looks porous and dull.

The second, cortex, layer, is where the pigment is stored and into which some chemicals penetrate. The outer scales lifted in the process of penetration are not always smoothed down again completely when you change hair colour or texture, and this causes porosity. The medulla, or innermost layer, is sometimes absent in very fine hair.

Both heat-styling and perming modify part of the hair structure to induce change in the shape of the hair and how it waves or curls. Hair colourants – the permanent variety using oxidation dyes – lift the hair's protective outer cuticle scales, too, to impart or change the pigment inside, while bleaching works by neutralising some of the darker natural pigment. The more we do to our hair – whether it is blow-drying, heat-styling, perming or colouring – the more likely it is to be porous, dry and dull. Pollution, smoke, sunlight and extremes of temperature also have an affect on hair, as do fashionable hairstyles. So haircare has to be a continuous process in order for your hair to look in peak condition.

Heat and chemicals make the hair lose moisture and – as so many of us heat-dry and style our hair, and have perms and colourants – it's no wonder that dry hair is becoming commonplace. Hair that dries out resists styling and is more difficult to manage. Think of your hair as a delicate and expensive yarn that needs to be pampered, rather like a luxurious cashmere sweater, and you'll be on the right track!

Caring for your hair means choosing the right shampoo and doing regular conditioning.

IN THE WASH

We are all washing our hair more often these days, hence the advent of the frequent-use shampoo. This is formulated not to strip away too much of the hair's natural oils which lubricate the hair, stop moisture loss, and help hair to be more manageable.

You can find shampoos specially for heat-styled or coloured hair, as well as for dry hair, and there are even some ranges especially for permed hair. If your hair is oily, use a frequent-use shampoo. Strong detergent shampoos for oily hair are now out of favour.

If you wash your hair a lot you may only need one lather-up, not two, and when you dry your hair afterwards, blot it with a towel, but don't rub. Wet hair tends to stretch and break and is very vulnerable so never use a bristle brush on hair when wet. Comb through with a wide-toothed comb that has rounded ends, or a wide-apart nylon-bristle styling brush.

Take the trouble to rinse your hair really thoroughly, especially round the hairline.

Keep the gloss
Conditioners reduce static and fly-away, smooth down lifted or damaged cuticle scales, and make hair easier to comb and style. Cream conditioners are massaged onto hair, left on for a few minutes, then rinsed off. But there are other forms of conditioning, too.

Intensive-care conditioners are often thick creams, and are meant to be used on damaged hair as and when you need it. Apply, comb through, put on a plastic bath cap to keep in the heat and leave on for about 20–30 minutes.

Spray-on hair glosses and hair dressings are meant to be used on dry hair in between shampoos and are particularly useful on coarse, curly hair that lacks moisture.

Hot-oil treatments are useful for permed, coloured, sun-dried or heat-dried hair, as a once-in-a-while extra. Warm up the oil in a cup, standing in hot water (either buy a sachet of hair treatment oil, or use almond oil). Afterwards, shampoo off.

HEALTHIER HAIRSTYLING

Any tool you use on your hair, be it hairdryer, curling tongs, brush or comb, can damage and tear, so choose carefully and use gently.

Heat drying can literally 'cook' the hair, so always hold your dryer at least 12 inches away from your head and keep it moving. Never concentrate the heat in one place for long.

Use the gentler heat if your dryer has variable adjustments. It may take longer but it helps to avoid damage. Try not to use heated rollers, styler or dryer every day. If you have the type of hair that can take it, try to leave hair to dry naturally, without heat, scrunching it with a little mousse. You may find that's all you need. When heat styling, use a vent brush which allows hot air to circulate through the brush, spreading the heat evenly.

Never use rubber bands to tie back your hair: it's a sure way to get hair breakage. It is worth buying covered elastic bands or using a ribbon.

PROBLEM SOLVING

Some of the following problems may be encountered by even the healthiest head of hair some time during its long and variously-styled life:

Dandruff

This is when scalp skin sheds excessively, leaving tiny flakes showing on hair and shoulders. It is very common and all kinds of reasons have been put forward to explain its occurrence – from stress to microbial attack.

Ordinary everyday flaking can be controlled with an anti-dandruff shampoo. Some of the best contain an ingredient called zinc pyrithione. Other shampoos contain sulphur and salicylic acid that may help. If you have the kind of problem that involves an inflamed, itchy, red scalp, with a rash spreading down onto forehead and behind the ears, do see your doctor. This could be seborrhoeic eczema and you may be recommended to use a tar shampoo.

Hair loss

We all lose some hair every day and that is normal. But excessive hair loss, in which hair falls out in handfuls, leaving you with thinner hair or bare patches, is more serious. You may lose hair because of illness or a shock, and it is common to have hair loss about three months after having a baby, but this is only temporary and the hair grows back.

During its growth phase (called *anagen*) hair grows for between three and six years, Then there is a short resting period (telogen) of about three months, when the hair is shed. Normally, about 85% of your hair is in the anagen phase and 15% in telogen.

But sometimes hair enters the telogen phase too early. There are different kinds of hair loss, some non-genetic. *Traction alopecia* is caused by tightly pulled pony-tails, braids and chignons; *friction alopecia* occurs when hair bands, wigs or hats are too tight and the hair breaks off. *Alopecia areata* is a disease of the scalp in which baldness is patchy and progressive.

In contrast, common male pattern baldness is influenced by age, heredity and the actions of androgens (male sex hormones) on the hair follicles. Some women, too, have the condition although there are no other signs of masculinity.

If you feel that you may be losing too much hair, do see your doctor, who may refer you to a special hair clinic. Sometimes hair grows back of its own accord. About one third of all cases recover after the first episode of *alopecia areata*, and never get another bald patch. Two-thirds may relapse within six months but there is still a good chance that the condition will clear up ultimately.

Broken and damaged hair

This is usually caused by ill-treatment with chemicals, heat or styling aids. Over-bleaching is a real hair-destroyer so do not embark on it lightly if you have dark hair. After long use of permanent hair colourants, which penetrate the hair shaft, hair may be porous, broken and dull.

So what can you do about it? Examine your methods. If you have the sort of hairstyle that shows up the root regrowth within three weeks, necessitating retouching with either bleach or colourant, consider a restyle. Smooth hair will show up roots – curly hair or hair with movement tends to disguise the roots. So you can go for longer without a tint.

Use a semi-permanent colour to disguise grey roots in between your permanent tint sessions. Semi-permanents that do not contain oxidation dyes just stain the outer hair and do not cause porosity and damage. They wash out over a number of shampoos.

Instead of whole-head bleach, consider streaking – then you don't have to have retouching so often.

Don't do so much heat-styling and drying. Let hair dry naturally as often as you can. Avoid rubber bands, spiky brushes and combs, and do cover up your hair in the sun. Use a good conditioner every time you shampoo.

SET WITH STYLE

Looking after your own hair at home has never been easier with the huge selection of style aids such as gels, mousses, creams, waxes and spray setters and finishers to choose from.

Use gel for sculptured, spiky or slicked back styles, or for crisping up fringes and pieces. It is useful for short hair, and can be fingered in wherever you need it.

Mousse is great for finger-drying, blow-drying or scrunch-drying. You can get a natural effect with regular-strength mousse or more control with the stronger varieties. It gives curly or permed hair more shape and less frizz, and gives style support for straight hair, reducing static, adding body and bounce.

Waxes and creams give shine and control for more structured styles. Fingered through permed or curly hair, they give more definition to curls and tendrils. Use sparingly.

Sprays are not just for keeping a finished style in place – they are useful for styling, too. For more body, spray the roots with head upside down, then toss the hair back. 'Structure' sprays are a sort of setting lotion in natural spray form, allowing permed or curly hair to be scrunched into shape.

COUNT ON COLOUR

Your choice of shade is very important if you want to change your hair colour. If you are going grey, don't try to recapture the dark brown you were 20 years ago. It could be far too hard – your skin tends to lose colour, too. Go for a couple of shades lighter – medium warm brown, for example, or dark blonde (sometimes known as light brown). Dense, dark, one-colour tinting is hard to take and looks false. Hair is naturally composed of lots of different tints, so streaking, lowlights and selected colouring gives a more flattering effect. Don't use a red shade of semi-permanent on hair that is mostly white – it might look too strident. Natural shades of mid- or lighter-brown are better.

Consider the cost of colour before you plunge. It is not just the initial charge but also the upkeep – permanently tinted or lightened hair will need the roots retouching regularly. The bigger the difference in shade between your own natural colouring and the new, the more your roots will show up.

The importance of a good hairdresser

Dressed hair is as important to the overall appearance as a well made-up face.

It was not until I met my current hairdresser (who thankfully is still in the same place three years later!) that I realised the importance of a good head of hair, stylishly cut, well-conditioned and subtly coloured. He has been instrumental in the complete change in my appearance – a good hairdresser is a very valuable asset! Take a look

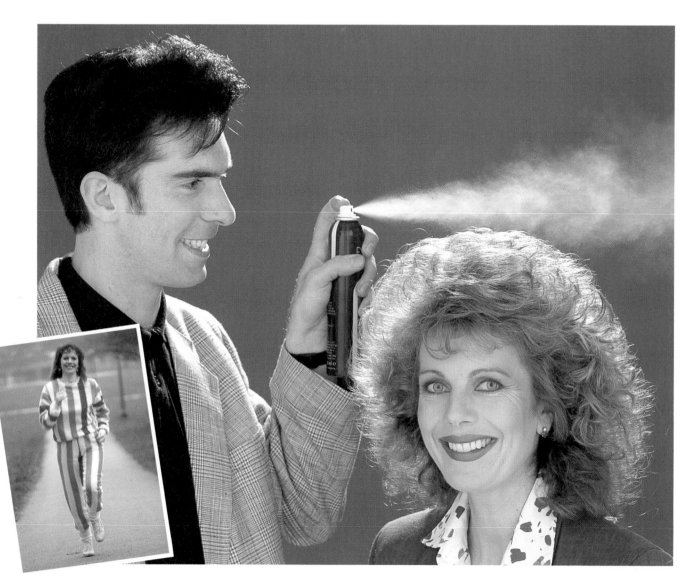

at the two photographs (above) and this will equally convince you that since being in the hands of an expert it really has become my 'crowning head of glory'.

For so long I resisted any change to my hairstyle – I thought *I* knew what suited me – I was entrenched in an image that I had held from years gone by. Do be *advised* by your hair-dresser. If he/she confidently can explain how a certain style will enhance your best features, then listen. After all, they deal with endless different-shaped heads all day long, coiffuring styles that emphasise a client's best features. Two heads may indeed be better than one! If you are prepared to be guided and be open to change, who knows? Your change of hairstyle may be a significant step in beginning to look a million dollars!

FINISHING TOUCHES

Cosmetics are beauty enhancers as well as camouflagers – what would we do without them! Whether you pay a little or a lot, it is your skill in applying make-up which matters, and anybody can learn to be their own best make-up artist.

Gone are the days when you had to wear cosmetic colours that matched your brows or hair. Now, it is permissible to wear all kinds of shades, according to your clothes as well as your personal colouring. Red-heads can and do wear pinks, as well as terracotta and greens. Brunettes can choose smokey greys and khakis as well as browns, and blondes do not have to wear blues all the time, even with blue eyes. Why not green, or even pinks and golds?

The secret of success is to experiment – on yourself. Only by trying out different colours and effects will you be able to find one that does the most for *your* looks.

In the Pink
Nothing flatters a post-winter pallor more than soft, skin-friendly pinks – nor makes the most of

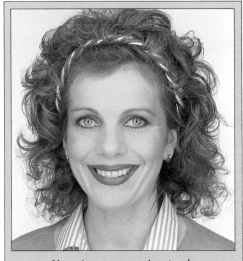
Use colour to your advantage!

a summer tan. Shades of wine and roses may be beauty staples, but they are major complexion enliveners nonetheless. They work for just about everybody, given the right choice of shade.

Soft buffs, blushes, corals, peach-pink tints or deep-set magentas – pinks are the most flattering set of colours. Use the darkest pinks on lids and lips, for example, then lightly highlight cheeks, chin and browbone with paler tones in the same family.

Compatible colours include teal, blueberry or moss, used as liner, mascara, or smudged over eyelids for a dramatic effect. Finish with a matt pink-toned lipstick applied with a brush for more accuracy and softness. Stronger pinks can be softened with brush-stroke application. They can be blotted down for an even more subtle finish, if you prefer, then topped with a dewy lipgloss.

If you like to wear gold jewellery, go for lighter, peachy pinks. If you prefer silver, stick with bluish pinks and deeper shades.
○ *Use* a foundation that closely matches your skintone, topped with transparent loose powder to set, then add your pinks. Use a fat blusher

brush to sweep a pinky blusher over cheekbones and to dust lightly over chin, browbone and perhaps temples.

Give your eyes a rosy touch with a rose-tinted eyeshadow on the browbone, to meet a subtle grey-brown in the socket. This gives eyes a more sculptured look. Use a touch of paler pink on lids, as long as they are not too prominent. Brush on golden brown or grey under lower lashes. Or use a blueberry-grey shade on lids, with matching smudgy line under lashes. Use a cotton bud to blend the colours together, so there are no hard lines.

Paint on your lip shape with a matching pink lip pencil, or use a brush with pink lipstick. Fill in both lips, then top the centre of the bottom lip with a touch of pinky lipgloss for a dewy finish.

Warm and Glowing

Wear sunlit shades to give your looks a lift – enhancing a tan, prolonging it, or to give yourself a slight sun-kissed healthy shimmer. This look is more vivid – a sunwarmed skin, lightly touched with gold, subtly shaded desert-flower eyes, and lips a clear, intense colour. This is a flattering look for medium blondes and brunettes.
○ *Use* a tinted moisturiser, or a moisturised base that is softly glowing, but do not use anything too different from your natural skintone or it will look unnatural. Be careful to blend away base or tinted moisturiser into the neck. Apply cream blusher in a soft terracotta shade, or powder first, then apply a powder blusher in glowing earthy tone.

Try lining the upper lids with a soft sage eye-contouring pencil. Then brush a subtle green across the entire lid. Apply a warm khaki-green on the browbone, rounding down to the outside corner of the eye, and highlight with an orangy glow just under the arch of the eyebrow. Apply a sunlit coral shade of lipstick – outline first with matching lip pencil.

Be a Shady Lady

This is the look for a fairly pale skin. Match base to your skin and top with translucent powder. Keep blusher soft and very gentle. Shaded, smokey eyes with a feeling of the 60's promise drama. Go for sludgy, smudgy shadows that eclipse the eye, giving shape and shade, dark thick lashes and structured brows.
○ *Use* grey-blues, taupes, khakis, subtle grey-browns, smokey subtle grey-purples. Blend the darker shadow outwards from the centre of the lid, leaving the inner eye paler. Blend and smudge the darker colours under the bottom lashes from the outer corner to the middle of the eye. Then use liner on the eyelids. Define brows with a brush and grey or brown eyeshadow or brow definer, or use a pencil softened with a brush. Let the eyes hold the spotlight and keep lips muted with soft pink or peach.

TIPS AND TRICKS

Here are some extra pointers to creating your perfect look:

Face

○ Use a stick or cream concealer under eyes to disguise dark circles, or try a touch of paler-toned foundation. Blend away the edges.
○ Disguise a blemish with a touch of medicated cover-stick, then set with loose face powder. Use a cotton bud to carefully blend away edges into foundation so there is no hard edge.
○ Do not use a brush straight from pot to face. Use your hand as a palette so you do not put on too much colour at one time.
○ Avoid sparkly foundations and powders unless your skin and features are very good. Shine draws the attention and tends to exaggerate. So if you want to camouflage a big feature, keep it matt. Careful application of a slightly darker foundation can slim a big nose.

○ Use a dampened sponge to apply foundation for a natural look and longer-lasting make-up.

○ Remember less is best if you are getting a bit older. Too thick make-up may accentuate wrinkles, and very bright and dark colours may look too garish.

○ Apply plenty of loose face powder if you want a make-up that lasts the day. Brush away surplus after application, using a big, soft powder brush. Do not leave too much sitting in laughter lines or they will seem like crevices!

○ Tone down high colouring by using a green moisturiser or under-make-up base before applying foundation. Or use concealer underneath. Just apply to the rosy parts and blend away the edges.

○ Sit in front of a good light when making-up. Do it in front of a window or take the shade from a table-lamp if necessary. Remember that make-up tones tend to change according to the lighting conditions – daylight is more blue, and electric light is more yellow.

○ Avoid a shiny nose – use a water-based matt or anti-shine foundation and plenty of loose powder.

Lips

○ To make thin lips look fuller, add a touch of lipgloss on the centre of the lower lip as a final touch.

○ Paler, shiny colours help thin lips look more full. It is not a good idea to go over the natural lipline – it usually looks false.

○ Use a deeper lip shade to make thick lips look slimmer – keep just inside the natural lipline.

○ Dry lips? Apply a lip moisturiser or lip balm about 20 minutes before you want to apply lipstick. Blot the surplus.

○ Apply foundation over your lips and then powder to give a good base for your lipstick.

○ For lips that stick, and a crisper outline (less ageing than a fuzzy one), outline lips with lip pencil in a shade that matches your lipstick. Fill in, blot on a tissue, then reapply another coat of lipstick.

Eyes

○ Avoid irridescent, pearly or sparkly shadows, if you have crepey, lined lids.

○ Reduce prominent lids with a matte, sludgy shade of eyeshadow over the entire lid, blended away up to the brow. Avoid frosted cosmetics and highlights on the lids. Use eyeliner because it tends to reduce the size of the lid above.

○ 'Bring out' deep-set eyes with a paler shadow – obviously darker tints will tend to shade the eye and make it look deeper.

○ Close-set eyes need the emphasis on the outer eye, swept up to brow. If you use liner, start from the centre lid. Try using a paler shadow at the inner corner of the lids and blend to a deeper tone on the outside.

○ Sparse eyebrows can be filled in with a sharpened eye pencil, but soften with a brush afterwards so there is no hard line. Do follow the natural shape – drawing in new eyebrows can make you look permanently surprised or over-made-up.

○ Take the trouble to have very fair lashes (and brows, if necessary) dyed. It is convenient for summer beauty – and good for older women. Darker lashes and brows make you look more wide-awake and add definition, even when you are not wearing other make-up.

○ Soften the effect of eyeliners by using a small-headed eyeliner brush with dark shadow, brushed subtly under lashes, or applied over liner to set it.

YOUR DAILY SESSION

Here's a step-by-step guide for making-up your face. I'm sure you have your own routine, but do try these basic rules which are well worthy applying. Over the years with the help of several experts I've learnt the secrets of the make-up artists: how to highlight the areas of the face that are assets and how to cover the less flattering features! Colours in fashion change, but the basic principles always apply.

DAY MAKE-UP

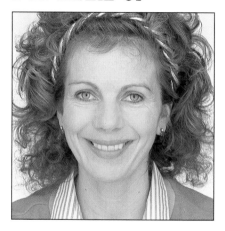 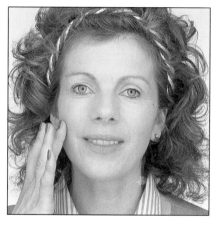 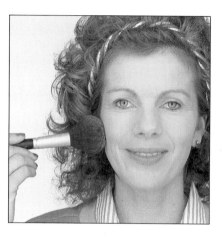

1 If it's possible, make-up by natural light and always start with a clean canvas!

2 **Foundation** To give a smooth appearance and to cover *all* flaws, spots, thread veins and any blemishes, gently tap on your foundation. Cover-up sticks or creams and lighteners are too heavy and are invariably a different colour from the foundation. Don't dot the foundation all over the face to begin with because it's difficult to gauge how much is needed. Use your fingers or a dampened sponge.

Finish by applying the foundation on the eyelids so it can be powdered immediately, preventing it from melting into creases.

3 Powder the rest of the face. Loose translucent powder is best, as it's much finer than pressed powder. Dust off any excess. This is not always necessary on liquid-based foundation as it dries and will set without leaving any residue.

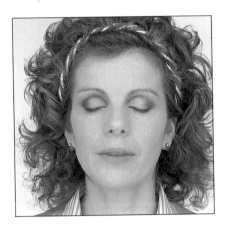

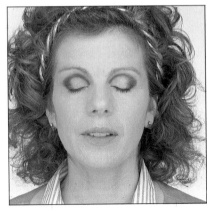

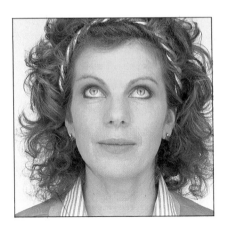

4 **The Eyes** Use a powder shadow as it blends well and stays best. A warm brown will enhance any eye colour. Apply under the socket bone and on the outer third of the lid, from lashes to socket. Lightly press on and don't rub.

5 To soften around the eyes, blend the edges of the eye shadow. Use a cotton wool bud for this. When applying eyeliner, try using a little water mixed with eye shadow powder – it gives a softer, less harsh, line.

6 For underneath the eyes, use a soft eye pencil – I use dark brown – starting thinly at the centre of the eye and taking it gradually thicker to the outer corner. Blend the edges into the eye line.

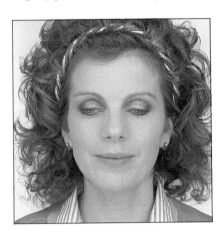

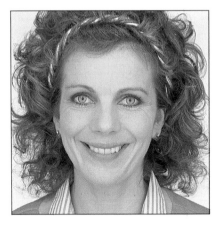

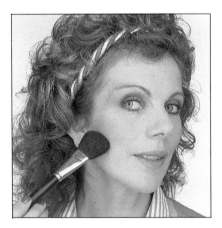

7 To the rest of the eyelid, apply peachy, bronze highlighter. Blend where the highlighter joins the socket shadow and outer third of the eyelid.

8 **Eyelashes and Eyebrows** Apply black mascara and separate lashes with a lash comb. Apply to your bottom lashes first – use the point of the mascara wand and work down lashes individually.

Darken the eyebrows with dark brown or black powder – pencil gives a very harsh look. Blend gently with a finger if necessary.

9 **Blusher** Foundation and powder take away the definition, so blusher will colour and shape the face.

Apply under the cheekbone, pushing upwards so that it goes slightly onto the bone. This will give the impression of a higher cheekbone. Draw an imaginary line from the centre of eye to under the cheekbone and start there, pushing upwards.

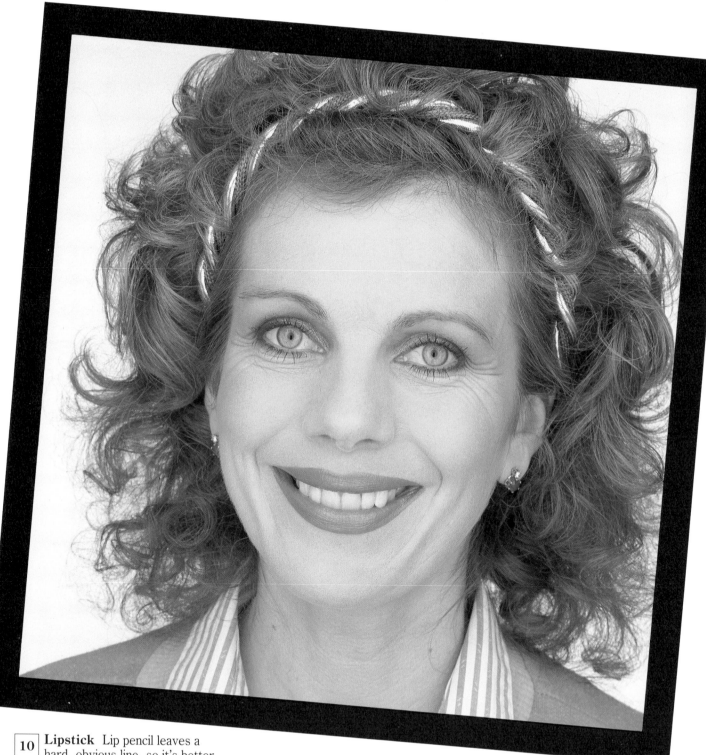

| 10 | **Lipstick** Lip pencil leaves a hard, obvious line, so it's better to use a brush. Work from the corner to the centre of the lips – first one side, then the other; top then bottom.

EVENING MAKE-UP

Cleansing and re-applying make-up can irritate the skin if you've been fully made up during the day. It is kinder and easier to the skin to freshen up your existing make-up, highlighting and exaggerating for the artificial light of night. Blend away any creases in your make-up and gently apply the new eyeshadow, highlighter and pencil, the blusher and lipstick.

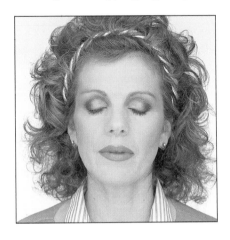

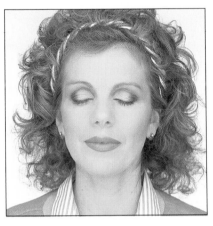

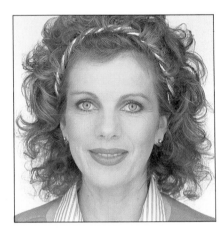

1 **The Eyes** Apply dark brown shadow over the socket and, as in day make-up, over one-third of the eye. Blend at the edges.

2 Apply slightly lighter highlighter on the remaining two-thirds of the eye – I prefer something with a little sparkle.

3 Draw the shadow pencil all the way under the lower lashes, from the inner corner to outer edge and just onto the upper lid. Blend.

4 Apply cream-coloured eye pencil – *not* white – onto the inner ridge of the lower lid. This will open eyes up and give bright, clear-looking eyes – especially late at night if you've got pink-rimmed tired eyes! Be careful, though, not to get it on eyelashes.

5 **Blusher** Slightly strengthen your blusher. Then apply the brush again on the brow bone over the eyebrow to hairline and bring around to join the blusher on cheeks.

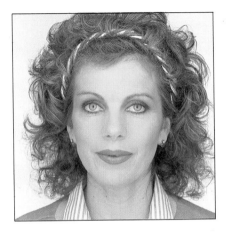

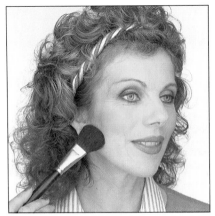

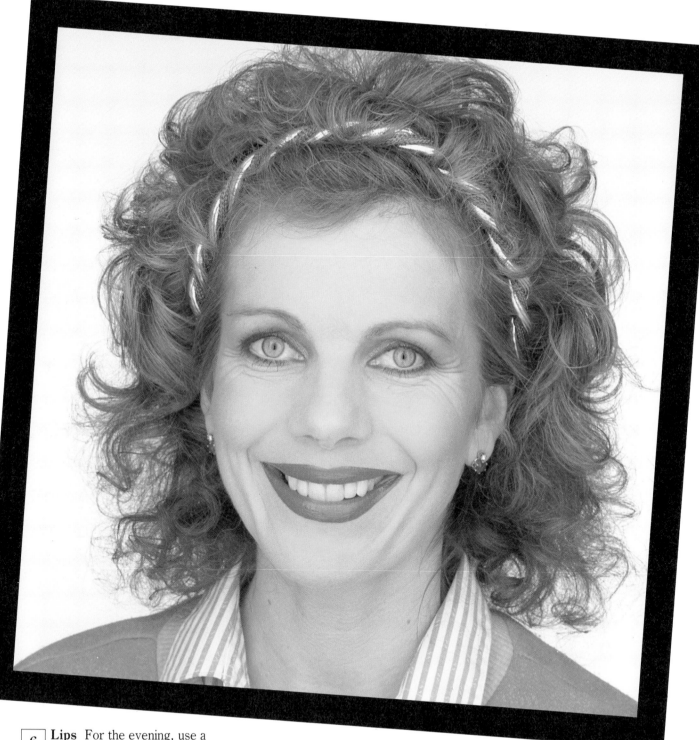

6 **Lips** For the evening, use a darker, brighter lip colour. (Blot and clean off your day colour.) Add a little gloss on the centre.

POISE and BODY LANGUAGE

Consider how you sit, stand and walk and remember that individuality, habits and inner feelings are expressed through movement.

Exercise will help your posture, improve your body awareness, give you greater confidence and fluidity of line and co-ordination when you move, particularly if you're wearing high heels. With regular exercise, you're half way there.

Now let's look at ourselves from top to toe and see what signals we are giving out. Body awareness can help to develop confidence, although you should never forget that we are all basically shy; it's just that some disguise is better than others. Practise all the tips in front of a full-length mirror at home.

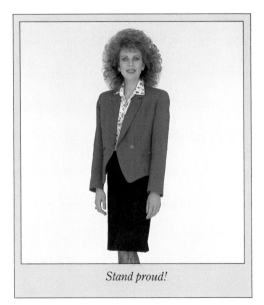

Stand proud!

HEAD ANGLE AND EYES

When you're feeling ill at ease, the head angle is difficult to control. This is because the eyes are truly 'the mirror of the soul' and even if we lie through our teeth they'll still give the game away.

We look at the floor and turn away shiftily to avoid confronting the person we are attempting to communicate with. The head is invariably inclined and we look up and out through the corner of an eye.

So, adjust the angle of your head and look straight into the eyes of the other person. If you find this impossible, choose the point between their eyes, at the top of the nose. You'll find this much easier.

And remember always to look into a person's eyes as you shake hands. It's only for a fleeting moment but shows strength.

SHOULDERS BACK

Tension collects around the base of the neck and shoulders and can help create the wrong body shape and signals. The answer is to do exercises that alleviate the tension.

The most common fault is the droop, which can be the result of inhibitions dating from your teens when your breasts formed, or simply an inability to face up to the world. Also, if you lead a stressful, fast-paced life and rarely relax, your shoulders become painfully tense.

Remember being told as a child, 'Don't slouch – sit up straight!'? Well, there was sound method in what seemed to be bullying.

ARMS AND HANDS

There's a wonderful play by N.F. Simpson, *The One Way Pendulum*, in which one of the characters repeatedly stands before the mirror and says, 'I can't go out with arms like these – they're too long.'

The more she looks at them, the longer they seem to become. Perhaps you know what she means. Sometimes you feel your arms are in the way, as they dangle awkwardly by your side. So what should you do with them?

Try standing with one hand in your pocket, or carry a clutch bag. Never fold your arms – it's a sign of aggression and can be misconstrued as an attempt to block somebody out.

And the hands? If you're standing, place both arms slightly in front of you, which will give the hands a gentle lock. That's what the Royal Family does. If you're sitting, the same rule applies, but place your hands in your lap and cup one lightly in the other. Don't fiddle or hold on to a ring tightly.

LEG LESSONS

When you are standing, hold your hands in front of you and keep your legs close together. The stance is firm and elegant. Pull up your leg muscles and you'll be steady as a rock.

When seated, you can often send out the wrong signal with the legs, real giveaways.

Don't cross your legs for lengthy periods, you'll inhibit the blood flow.

Don't entwine them. You look as though you're

holding on to yourself for security.

Don't be a leg flapper (something I have to control). There's nothing more distracting than watching a crossed leg going up and down in an incessant rhythm.

Don't sit with your legs wide apart even when wearing trousers. Look at the pictures and you'll see there are two ideal sitting positions. Place one foot a little in front of the other and slightly apart. Or tuck one behind the other so both legs are at an angle. This can look extremely elegant. And if you have big legs, don't squash them together.

Make fashion work for you, enjoy it, just like the stars do.

CENTRE POINTS

Your centre strength is in your back and stomach. Again, exercise will help the posture in an area that is important to poise, both in sitting and walking.

Control those tummy muscles at all times, getting used to pulling them in. Who needs a girdle when you can do the work yourself?

Too often, exercise is thought of in isolation, for the class or dance studio. But you can exercise almost anywhere.

Always strengthen the back; don't hollow it or you'll throw your spine out of alignment and stick out your bottom. The result will not only be bad posture, but also eventual back pain, particularly in the lumbar region.

FILL YOUR SPACE

Hemmed in by the pressures of everyday living, we get 'crushed' into ourselves. So reach out every so often, take your arms out to your sides and remind yourself that all that space is yours.

GENERAL INDEX

RECIPE INDEX